Reviews of *Valley Fever Epidemic*

"The authors have filled a need for a detailed understanding of San Joaquin Valley Fever (Coccidioidomycosis) aimed at the patient, their families and their caregivers. This volume reflects the extensive research done by them and their ability to convey this information. This volume is complete, up to date and accurate in describing this illness, the difficulties in diagnosis, treatment and vagaries of outcomes are well discussed."

Hans Einstein, MD, FACP
World's Foremost Valley Fever Expert and Treatment Pioneer
Bakersfield, California

"I am a board-certified Infectious Disease physician, and have treated more than 2500 patients with severe *Coccidioides* infection over the past 19 years, both here in Arizona and previously in Texas.

"*Valley Fever Epidemic* offers a good overview of the spectrum of disease associated with this pathogen. It includes discussion of the problems that patients may face with misdiagnosis and drug therapy for the disease. The section 'Helpful Hints for Your Doctor Visits' would be good reading for any patient, no matter what their problems."

Steven L. Oscherwitz, MD
Diplomate, American Board of Internal Medicine and Infectious Diseases
Tempe, Arizona

Reviews of *Valley Fever Epidemic*

"Sharon and David Filip's book *Valley Fever Epidemic* is a comprehensive review of the fungus 'cocci' that has been so devastating to those who visit and live in the region where this fungus exists, primarily Arizona and California. This book covers everything from cause to treatment as well as the harsh eye opening reality of those people and pets who suffer with this sometimes elusive disease. They delicately bring out the enigmatic reality of the lack of support for vaccine development and new drugs to prevent and treat this disease known for over 100 years. This is a valuable, well researched book and I would highly recommend it for patients, their family members, endemic area residents, and tourists."

Dr. Craig M. Rundbaken, DO, FCCP, FACOI
Pulmonary/Valley Fever Clinic
Sun City West, Arizona

"Fulfils with consummate ease the authors' aim of providing a comprehensive guide to coccidioidomycosis for patients and families. Immaculately researched and presented in language accessible to the lay reader with a dedicated glossary to facilitate understanding of medical literature. Culminates in a call to arms to support development of a preventive vaccine and curative pharmacotherapy, while itself holding the potential to raise awareness of this under-diagnosed disease among health care providers."

Dr Srijita Sen-Chowdhry MA, MBBS, MRCP, MD (Cantab.)
Cardiologist
London, UK

Reviews of *Valley Fever Epidemic*

"Thank you for presenting this remarkable compilation of facts and personal stories about Valley Fever. This is a disease that many would just as soon sweep under the rug—you've laid the dust out where all can see! Victims of severe cases of Valley Fever will want their family, friends and business associates to read this book to better understand this so often 'invisible' disease affecting their lives. There are many working very hard to find a vaccine. Perhaps this book will explain to those who haven't yet been touched personally by the disease why the vaccine effort is important to everyone."

Sandra Larson
Executive Director, Valley Fever Americas Foundation and the Valley Fever Vaccine Project of the Americas: A Rotary District 5240 Project

"This book is a layman's comprehensive review of the nature and treatment of Valley Fever. It provides the reader with an understanding of the endemic regions of the disease, factors which contribute to the incidence of Valley fever in humans and pets, and symptoms of the respiratory infection. The authors have provided useful resources in the form of web sites and scientific publications which readers can access for additional information on diagnosis and treatment of this insidious disease. A particularly appealing section of the book is devoted to personal accounts of individuals who survived infection with the Valley Fever pathogen. Many of these stories will be an inspiration to victims of the disease. A major goal of the authors was to elevate the level of awareness of potential complications of Valley Fever among both the resident population and those who visit the endemic regions of southwestern United States. In this regard, the message was clearly presented."

Garry T. Cole, PhD
Professor of Biology
Margaret Batts Tobin Endowed Chair
Department of Biology, University of Texas at San Antonio
World Leading Valley Fever Vaccine Researcher

Reviews of *Valley Fever Epidemic*

"I am overwhelmed and thrilled that someone has FINALLY written a book about Valley Fever. You have done an unbelievably outstanding job researching this subject, and I found the book to be extremely enlightening, easy to read and easy to understand.

"More importantly, this book has vindicated me and many others afflicted with Coccidioidomycosis, who have been ridiculed and told to 'get a life,' as well as others who have been forced to go from doctor to doctor because the medical profession, as a whole, does not recognize the severity of this disease.

"Had this book been available when I was first diagnosed, it would not have taken me over a year, and several doctors, and many tests, to finally find the right doctor. It would have spared me all the days and nights of tears and fear over what to do and worry over why no one believed me.

"Your six years of hard work have paid off with this wonderful achievement.

"I thank you."

Honey De Serre, Editor
The Bugler & The Sentinel
Publications of the Jewish War Veterans (JWV) of the USA
Copper State Post 619 & Dep't of Southwest

What others are saying about Valley Fever

"We appreciate your continued advocacy for public awareness."

Julie Louise Gerberding, MD, MPH, Director of the Centers for Disease Control and Prevention (CDC) in her letter to Sharon Filip and David Filip.

"Valley Fever is a grossly underdiagnosed disease, and doctors need to think about it early, not late."

Mark Wright, Clinical Assistant Professor in the University of Arizona Department of Emergency Medicine, Medical Director of the Urgent Care Center.

"...we who live and breathe here in the major epicenter of the disease are at risk of dying of it. There is no cure...When disseminated throughout the body, valley fever can cause extreme pain, stiffness, mental debility, paralysis and death."

Bakersfield Californian Editorial Staff

"The incidence of disease has been increasing with the expansion of city borders. Disease prevalence is now stretching across the globe due to rising tourist industries in endemic areas with high visitation rates by foreign travelers...the prevalence and distribution of coccidioidomycosis is increasing as is the likelihood of seeing its often unique and bizarre clinical manifestations and complications."

Lewicky YM, Roberto RF, Curtin SL. The unique complications of coccidioidomycosis of the spine: a detailed time line of disease progression and suppression. Spine. 2004 Oct 1;29(19):E435-41.

What others are saying about Valley Fever

"People don't understand that this disease in this country actually kills more people per year than does tuberculosis. [Valley Fever] has a significant public health burden that is not really appreciated."

Dr. Richard Hector
Project Director, Valley Fever Vaccine Project

"A lot of people thought the only way to get sick is to be around construction sites or places with a lot of dust. The truth is there's a lot of dust in Arizona in general, so if you breathe here, you can catch it."

Jose Miguel, KNXV ABC 15
Phoenix, Arizona

"What I'm seeing are much more severe cases — dogs with insidious complications that are not responding to medications. I just can't seem to make them well."

Dr. Lisa Shubitz, DVM
Phoenix, Arizona

"Arizona is seeing a rising number of infections, a trend that alarms and puzzles state health officials...Because Valley fever is considered a possible bioterror agent, along with anthrax and smallpox, it's time for the Departments of Homeland Security and Defense to ante up."

Arizona Republic Editorial Staff.

Valley Fever
Epidemic

Valley Fever
Epidemic

David Filip and Sharon Filip

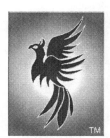

Golden
Phoenix
Books

Published in July 2008 by Golden Phoenix Books

http://www.goldenphoenixbooks.com
http://www.valleyfeversurvivor.com
http://www.valleyfeverepidemic.com

Publisher's Cataloging in Publication Data

Filip, David.
   Valley fever epidemic / by David Filip and Sharon Filip
   p. cm.
   Includes bibliography, glossary, and index.
   ISBN 978-0-9798692-5-9 (alk. paper)
1. Coccidioidomycosis—Popular works.   2. Coccidioidomycosis—
Dictionaries.   3. Coccidioidomycosis—Bibliography.
   I. Filip, Sharon. II. Title.
RC136.3.F55 2008
616.969—dc22

Library of Congress Control Number: 2008904803

Printed in the United States of America on acid-free paper.

Dedication

This book is dedicated to all those who are presently suffering with Valley Fever, their families, and all those yet to come who will fall ill to this incurable and deadly disease.

This book was created out of the love, friendship and requests of many of our valleyfeversurvivor.com readers. We consider the Valley Fever community an extended part of our family. We have often heard complaints that Valley Fever patients did not receive adequate care or information from their doctors and had a painful lack of understanding from their families, friends, and co-workers.

The authors believe the best way to help patients, doctors, and families understand Valley Fever and obtain the best of care is to have the most important information available at their fingertips.

Acknowledgements

Sharon and Dave thank our family, Stan and Seth, for their editing expertise and for supporting us in the long hours we have dedicated volunteering for the Valley Fever community.

We want to thank Dr. Steven Oscherwitz, Dr. Craig Rundbaken, Dr. Srijita Sen-Chowdhry, Sandra Larson, and Dr. Garry Cole for taking the time to read *Valley Fever Epidemic*, offer suggestions, and write book reviews. We thank them all for their dedication to public health. We also thank Honey De Serre (a professional editor of two papers and a Valley Fever Survivor) for writing a review from a survivor's perspective. We thank Dr. Hillel B. Levine, Dr. John W. Rippon, Dr. David Ellis, and the University of Adelaide for permitting us to use their pictures.

The authors were especially thankful that Dr. Hans Einstein reviewed our book. We also want to honor him for his tireless work on Valley Fever. Dr. Einstein is a living legend and the world's foremost medical expert on Valley Fever, with over half a century of experience fighting this disease. He pioneered the use of intrathecal amphotericin B, the first effective way to fight meningitis caused by Valley Fever, worked on the vaccine project, and produced a large body of work in the medical journals at a time when information was scarce. Among his many credits include being president and fellow of many national and regional professional medical organizations as well as being a consultant and reviewer for various prestigious medical journals. Dr. Einstein continues staying active in the medical community and as an international consultant and educator to this day, with numerous honors and awards to his name. We are very appreciative that he gave of his time to review this book.

We thank our Valley Fever Survivor Support Group Directors Beverly Lobenstein, Linda Evins, Barbara Crummitt and Patricia White for their willingness to help others. A special thanks to Linda and Beverly and their families for their hard work on Valley Fever Survivor's first Vaccine Benefit, and to all of the www.valleyfeversurvivor.com readers who responded with surveys, questionnaires, and their experiences.

Table of Contents:

Introduction 1

Valley Fever Fundamentals... 7
ENDEMIC AREA MAPS AND INFORMATION.............................11
THE FIRST CASE...14
The Ongoing Significance of Early Discoveries 14

Statistics and Comparisons..16
ARIZONA STATISTICS 16
Hospital Cost Comparisons 16
CALIFORNIA STATISTICS 18
VALLEY FEVER VS. TUBERCULOSIS 18

Symptoms.. 20
SIGNS OF VALLEY FEVER 20
COMMON AND UNDIAGNOSED SYMPTOMS..............................22
A Frightening Example..22
WHY VALLEY FEVER'S SYMPTOMS MAKE DIAGNOSIS
DIFFICULT..22
SYMPTOMS IN ANIMALS 23

Risk Factors 24
VALLEY FEVER AT WORK 24
VALLEY FEVER AT PLAY...26
PERSONAL RISK FACTORS 27
Men at Risk..28
Pregnancy...28
Race...29
Age...32
Immune System Health 33
Smoking...35
Alcohol..35
Corticosteroids and Hormones 35

Other Drugs 36

Blood Type 37

Organ Transplants 37

Blood Transfusions: A Risk Factor? 37

Poverty 37

Frequently Asked Questions 38

Family: The Other Victims of Valley Fever 51

VALLEY FEVER AND FAMILY BREAKDOWNS 51

CHILDREN WITH VALLEY FEVER 54

CONFLICT OUTSIDE THE FAMILY 55

DEPRESSION 57

HOW PEOPLE CAN BE AFFECTED 58

AN IMPORTANT MESSAGE FOR FAMILY AND FRIENDS OF

EVERY VALLEY FEVER SURVIVOR 62

What You Need to Know Before You See a Doctor 67

AT A GLANCE 67

RISKS ASSOCIATED WITH SOME TESTS AND TREATMENTS 67

The Danger of Spinal Taps 68

Learn from Experience with Spinal Taps 69

Dangerous Radiation from CT Scans 70

MRI Dangers 72

HELPFUL HINTS FOR YOUR DOCTOR VISITS 74

Meet the Staff 74

Prepare your Questions 74

Request Copies of All Your Records 75

Protection Against the Cancer Misdiagnosis 76

Ask About Sanitation Procedures 77

Ask About the Lab Facilities 78

Beware of Drug Interactions 78

Keep a Critical Eye on Your Prescription 78

Take Charge 79

RELUCTANCE TO DIAGNOSE VALLEY FEVER 79

FRUSTRATION WITH MISDIAGNOSIS AND MEDICAL CARE 80

A PERSONAL MESSAGE FROM SHARON 83

Testing and Diagnosis **85**

AT A GLANCE..85
THE IMPORTANCE OF A VALLEY FEVER DIAGNOSIS..............85
UNDERSTANDING ANTIBODY TESTS FOR VALLEY FEVER 86
    Immune System Issues..88
    Complement Fixation Titers 89
    Other Antibody Tests 90
    ELISA Tests 92
    EIA Tests..92
    Immunodiffusion Tests 93
    Tube Precipitin..93
    Latex Agglutination 93
    Lab Lingo..93
    A Quick Review 95
    Quick Facts About Antibody Tests 96
OTHER METHODS OF DIAGNOSIS FOR VALLEY FEVER 96
    Biopsies, Samples, and Cultures 96
    Testing a Cultured Specimen 98
    Skin Tests...98
SUPPLEMENTAL TESTING 99
    Imaging Tests 99
    Erythrocyte Sedimentation Rate Tests 99
    Eosinophil Count Tests 100

Drugs and Treatment.. **101**

AT A GLANCE..101
SURGERY 101
DRUG BASICS..103
A SUMMARY OF DRUGS CURRENTLY USED FOR VALLEY
FEVER 104
AMPHOTERICIN B 104
AZOLE DRUGS 107
    Ketoconazole..108
    Itraconazole 109
    Fluconazole...110
    Azoles Vs. Amphotericin B......................................110

A NEW GENERATION OF ANTIFUNGAL DRUGS.....................111
    Posaconazole..111
    Voriconazole..112
    Caspofungin...113
THE VACCINE AND CURE PROJECTS.........................113
    The Valley Fever Vaccine Project..........................114
    The UTSA Vaccine Research..................................115
    Nikkomycin Z...116
    Roadblocks...116
DRUG INTERACTIONS..117
DOSAGE ISSUES...118
EASING THE EXPENSE..119
    Samples...119
    Valuable Insurance Information.............................119
    Pharmaceutical Philanthropy................................120
    Veterinary Assistance...121
    Tips for Buying Medicine.......................................122

Beyond Medical Care.. 123

AT A GLANCE..123
STRESS AND THE IMMUNE SYSTEM...........................123
THE ALKALINE DIET CONCEPT................................123
PROBIOTICS...125
MUSHROOMS FOR THE IMMUNE SYSTEM.....................126
INFLAMMATION...127
ANTIOXIDANTS..128
PHYSICAL THERAPY...130
    Raising Your Body Temperature.............................131
AN UNPROVEN AND DANGEROUS SELF-REMEDY.............132

Valley Fever in Animals... 134

WHAT TO LOOK FOR...134
MEDICAL CARE..135
STATISTICS..136
OCCURRENCES IN OTHER ANIMALS...........................136
STORIES OF ANIMALS WITH VALLEY FEVER..................137

Stories from Valley Fever Survivors........................ 148

SURVIVORS IN THEIR OWN WORDS............................149

The Future **171**

THE NEED FOR ACTION 173

OUR WORK CONTINUES 175

Appendix A: Organizations and Internet Resources 177

VALLEY FEVER ADVOCACY AND RESEARCH
ORGANIZATIONS 177

OTHER GROUPS OF INTEREST 180

Appendix B: Essential Facts 182

Appendix C: Glossary 195

Bibliography 231

Index of Drugs and Tests 250

Introduction

Have you ever been a visitor to or resident of Arizona, California, Texas, New Mexico, Nevada, Utah, Mexico, Central America, or South America?

Have you ever attended a university, sporting event, convention, or simply passed through any of these areas?

Did you get ill within one to four weeks after arriving home?

Do you currently have arthritis, rheumatism, chronic fatigue, fibromyalgia, respiratory infections or more?

If you answered yes to any of these questions, you may already be infected with the Southwest's incurable disease and not even know it.

Valley Fever is nothing new. Scientifically known as coccidioidomycosis, it is an insidious disease caused by the inhalation of airborne *Coccidioides* fungal spores (arthroconidia) released from arid soil in the Desert Southwest region of the United States. Internationally this fungus is also endemic to northern Mexico and parts of Central America and South America. This parasitic fungal disease is neither rare nor benign.

Valley Fever was first discovered near the turn of the 20th century, but became increasingly important as more and more people started to move to the area. The significance of Valley Fever has increased with the migration from Dust Bowl areas during the Great Depression, the training of the Army Air Corps during World War II, and the presently ongoing population boom in the Southwest. Valley Fever has plagued mankind long before it had been discovered by science, as evidenced by the discovery of thousand year-old Native American bones that had clearly been attacked by the fungus. It has been a part of the Desert Southwest for centuries, but its threat to public health could be ended if the vaccine and cure projects are funded to completion.

When most people hear the word "fungus" they usually consider it a simple annoyance like Athlete's Foot. They imagine they can take a pill or salve to get rid of a fungal infection and go on about their lives. That is far from reality with coccidioidomycosis in the human or animal body. *Coccidioides* replicates at such an alarming rate that it is considered the most virulent fungal parasite known to man.[72]

Further, *Coccidioides* is regulated along with anthrax and other biological weapons as a Select Agent in the Antiterrorism and Effective Death Penalty Act of 1996 and the Public Health Security and Bioterrorism Preparedness and Response Act of 2002. The Select Agent list is used in antiterrorism legislation and is reserved for toxins and biological agents "that have the potential to pose a severe threat to public health and safety."[43]

In a December 2007 letter attempting to appropriate funds for the Valley Fever Vaccine Project, U.S. Representative Kevin McCarthy of California stressed the importance of Valley Fever. He mentioned that the disease can be disabling, that drugs frequently fail to treat it, and that there are other horrors of the disease. "It is also important to note that between 200 and 500 people die annually from Valley Fever."[172]

This letter was co-signed by nine other U.S. Representatives: Devin Nunes, Ken Calvert, Jim Costa, George Radanovich, Darrell Issa, Rick Renzi, Raul Grijalva, Stevan Pearce, and Jon C. Porter.

When it comes to this particular fungal parasite, you should forget whatever you have heard about any other type of fungus, and even what you thought you knew about the fungus that causes Valley Fever.

No other fungus is regulated so heavily. It is considered so dangerous that the Centers for Disease Control (CDC), the Department of Health and Human Services, and the National Institutes of Health tell scientists culturing it in a laboratory to use Biosafety Level Three (BSL3) protocols and equipment.[120] These procedures are only one step below the maximum possible safety precautions that are reserved for the infamous hemorrhagic fever virus Ebola and other contagious diseases capable of causing biological catastrophes.

Of course, even with the strictest bioterrorism laws and laboratory regulations, people can still inhale *Coccidioides* any day of the year in Arizona, California, and other parts of the Southwest where it grows naturally. These are known as *endemic areas* to Valley Fever.

Valley Fever can be contracted easily because everyone needs to breathe. For this reason, everyone needs to know what this disease can do. Valley Fever can affect anyone from the unborn child to the great grandparent. It is a major problem for many animals as well. It is important for family, friends, and co-workers to understand what people with this disease are going through and ultimately to know what having this disease for a lifetime can mean.

In this book we tell everyone what they need to know to understand Valley Fever, how to get the best medical care, and how to be proactive in their health care after being infected with Valley Fever. It is written in easy to understand language with information that gets straight to the point so that everyone can learn the basics about Valley Fever, what it is, how and where it is contracted, and what the consequences are of being infected.

If you want to learn more, our facts are backed by hundreds of medical journal citations that provide important references for further research. To understand these documents or your own medical documentation, our comprehensive glossary will help you cut through the medical jargon. This is the first and only glossary ever created with the Valley Fever patient in mind.

Even if you never visit the Southwest, this information is still important to know because of Valley Fever transmission by fomites. Fomites are objects such as clothing, packing materials, fruits and vegetables, or virtually anything that can carry *Coccidioides* spores out of the endemic zones. Since fomites can be shipped anywhere in the world, this can cause a problem anywhere.

- A mechanic was "totally disabled" from cocci after working under a truck that had driven through endemic areas.[170]
- Cotton factory workers in Japan[189] and non-endemic parts of the United States[103] were sickened (with some fatalities) in outbreaks of Valley Fever due to *Coccidioides* spores brought to them on cotton.
- Iranian soldiers who had purchased American clothing were infected.[17]
- A 23-year-old steam boat crewman who had not been to endemic areas was found with Valley Fever lesions in both lungs and osteomyelitis, ultimately requiring the amputation of both feet.[211]

- A woman in Europe became infected with Valley Fever because someone mailed her a cactus from Arizona as a gift. *Coccidioides* spores were later found inside its pot.[27]
- A European traveler to Africa and Asia was also sickened. His doctors believed his dose of *Coccidioides* spores might have been "harboured in the air-conditioning system of an aircraft arriving from an endemic area" since the man had never visited North or South America, let alone the specific endemic areas.[193]

These and similar cases only tend to be noticed due to the "high mortality"[211] of cases related to fomite transmission, but there have been no major studies to determine what percentage of overall Valley Fever infections are due to fomites. Since many fomites are related to agriculture and California's fertile San Joaquin Valley is so hyperendemic to the disease that it is the origin of the name "Valley Fever," there is no vested interest for the local agricultural businesses and exporters to investigate how often and severely they might be spreading the disease.

This book is for everyone who lives in an endemic zone to *Coccidioides*, is or was a tourist there, or is considering visiting, going to school, working, retiring or relocating themselves and their family there. It has the comprehensive, basic facts that everyone needs to know *now*. This book will also benefit medical professionals with the latest, most accurate diagnosis and treatment information.

Please read all the information and check out all the peer reviewed medical journal citations in the book. With the knowledge and education you will receive from this book you will be able to decide what health risks you are willing to take for yourself, your spouse and children, your aging parents, and your beloved pets.

This book will highlight the specific risk factors for this disease. In addition it will note and dispel many misconceptions. For example, it is repeatedly stated in medical literature that seniors in particular are at risk. While this appears to be true *per capita*, it is also important to note that some data has shown people of other age groups to have cases reported more frequently. In Los Angeles County in 2006, the most frequently infected age group was 15-34 years old, and the second most infected age group was 45-54 years old.[166]

Also, many medical journal reviews of Valley Fever focus extensively on simple and asymptomatic Valley Fever cases. Not only does this undermine the seriousness of the illness to the populace at large, but many patients with life-threatening cases have been ignored or dismissed by doctors who were led to believe aggressive treatment would not be necessary.

In 2006, $50,000 in emergency funds were spent by the state of Arizona to educate doctors about Valley Fever. Even though that state is the heart of America's endemic areas, the need for education about this disease is critical for both the public and the medical community.

Medical professionals clearly need this information, both inside and outside the endemic regions. This book is invaluable to medical personnel to quickly learn the basics about Valley Fever, what it is, how it is treated, and ultimately how to help the patients that depend on them.

There were 8,916 Valley Fever cases reported nationally to the Centers for Disease Control in 2006. Since 2% or less of all Valley Fever infections are believed to be diagnosed correctly or diagnosed at all,[19, 244] that equates to an estimate of 445,000 people contracting this incurable disease in 2006. Strictly applying the 2% estimate to the 8,916 reported cases for 52 weeks or 365 days suggests 8,573 people each week or 1,221 people each day contracted Valley Fever in 2006.

All of these infections are unacceptable, whether the 2% of infections that were diagnosed or the 98% of the people that were misdiagnosed or undiagnosed. 2007 was nearly as severe, estimated to have produced nearly 400,000 new Valley Fever infections.

Naturally, the people behind these numbers are more important than any statistic. That is why this book features extensive quotations from the communication people had with www.valleyfeversurvivor.com in e-mails, questionnaires, and our online forums. It is not only the people who suffer with Valley Fever who contacted us, but also the family members who watch their loved ones lose their lives or have their quality of life deteriorate, and the pet owners who watch their beloved animal companions suffer and die.

We have included just a small sampling of the thousands of stories we have received. Sometimes people ask questions, sometimes they want to share information to help others avoid certain medical pitfalls, and sometimes they just want to vent their frustrations. While some stories included in this book have minor edits for spelling, grammar, and length, they appear nearly exactly as we had received them. The information they share tells more about the disease than you can read anywhere else.

If you have ever flown to, driven through, lived in or visited any region endemic to this disease, especially in Arizona or the San Joaquin Valley of California, you owe it to yourself and your family to thoroughly read this book. With awareness comes action, first to protect your loved ones, and ultimately to reach the goal of a vaccine and cure. Your health and lives may depend upon it.

Valley Fever Fundamentals

Valley Fever is the common name for the disease coccidioidomycosis, which is pronounced "cox-idd-ee-oy-doh-my-co-sis."

Although it has the name "Valley Fever" (shortened from "San Joaquin Valley Fever"), it should not be confused with and is completely unrelated to the Rift Valley Fever virus that occurs in Africa and the Middle East. Coccidioidomycosis is caused by fungi of the genus *Coccidioides* and is also frequently called "cocci" for short.

Coccidioides starts out as a fungus growing in the soil as mycelia (fibrous strands) made up of hyphae (branching tubes). Its microscopic appearance is often described as a "branching chain." Like many other fungi, they are saprobic, meaning that they feed off dead and decaying matter in the soil. This fungus does not produce a mushroom, is often underground, and looks like a mold when actually visible. The fungus is so tiny and so rarely produces a large mold that it is almost always invisible to the naked eye.

The reproductive spores called arthroconidia come off the fungus and are often picked up by the wind or other soil disturbances. While the mycelia are still microscopically small, the arthroconidia are even smaller, with a barrel shape that is approximately 2 micrometers wide by 4 micrometers long.[127] A micrometer (or micron) is one thousandth of a millimeter in length. Arthroconidial *Coccidioides* spores are roughly the same size as anthrax spores.

When a person or an animal inhales the *Coccidioides* arthroconidia, they may contract this incurable disease. In the lung the arthroconidia transform into round parasitic spores called spherules. *Coccidioides* is a dimorphic fungus, meaning it changes its form from a branching chain fungus in the ground to a spherically-shaped parasite in the body of its host.

The physical change in the fungus also signals a change in its behavior. As a saprobe it fed on organic matter in the soil. As a parasite it feeds on you (or any other infected human or animal host).

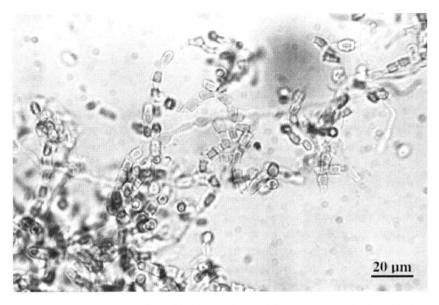

20 µm

A microscopic image of *Coccidioides* arthroconidia, courtesy Dr. David Ellis and the University of Adelaide.

It is not known why this fungus changes from a soil saprobe to a parasite. The transformation to its spherule form has been described in a medical conference as "being forced to transmutate, like nothing so much as the Hulk of television and comic strip fame, albeit with presumably less anger, to a totally new life form."[130]

Although they eat the person they infect, in a sense, *Coccidioides* spherules do not have teeth. They consume their host with chemical reactions that can lead to the destruction of soft tissue, bones, and nearly any organ. The spherule is 10-100 micrometers in diameter, but has yet another surprise in store.[215] As the spherule reaches maturity, it swells and ultimately breaks open, releasing between 200 and 1,000 endospores.[127, 217]

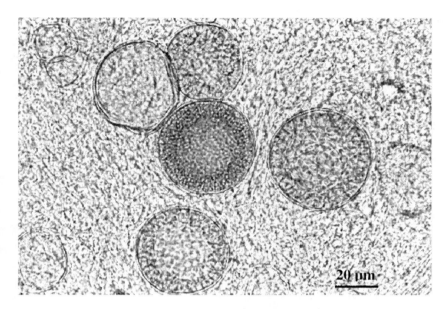

Coccidioides spherules with endospores inside and cultured from a lesion, as seen under a microscope.   Image courtesy Dr. David Ellis and the University of Adelaide.

Endospores are another tiny round form of this fungus, and have been found to be as small as 2 micrometers and as large as 10 micrometers in size while still contained within the maternal spherule.[127, 217]   Endospores are eventually released when the maternal spherule ruptures. Then they grow to become full size second generation spherules, thus repeating the life cycle from spherule to endospore again and again inside the host's body.

Since each spherule can produce so many endospores, Valley Fever can spread within the infected lung or to other organs of the body at an alarming rate.[153]   With a rapidly expanding population of fungal parasites working to eat their victim alive, it is easy to see how this fungal infection can be devastating in even the healthiest person or animal.

To complete the life cycle, if a person or animal dies from Valley Fever and the body decomposes in hot, dry soil with an occasional chance for moisture in endemic areas, the parasitic cells can transform back to saprobic mycelia and start this process over again.[152]

The Morphology of *Coccidioides* spp.

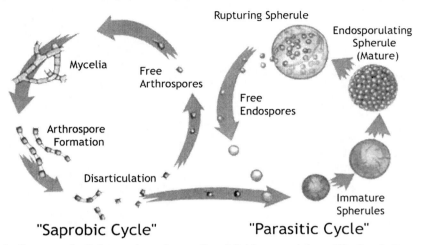

A diagram of all the various forms *Coccidioides* can take. We thank Dr. Hillel B. Levine for granting permission to use his life cycle artwork, and also for his pioneering work on Valley Fever. Dr. Levine is the creator of the original spherulin skin test.

Coccidioides immitis, often shortened to *C. immitis* is found in California. It is the most famous species of *Coccidioides* fungi due to the use of its name across a century of medical literature. By 2002, *Coccidioides posadasii* was finally considered to be a distinct species of the genus *Coccidioides.*[92] It has been called the "non-California" species of *Coccidioides* since *C. immitis* has been found only in California, and *C. posadasii* has been shown to have a wide geographical distribution through other parts of the United States, Mexico, Central America, and South America.[34]

Virtually all Valley Fever-related documentation before 2002 refers to *C. immitis,* especially since medical data were built on the belief that all strains were *C. immitis.* Sometimes the literature mentions *C. immitis* exclusively in the description of all *Coccidioides* fungi. As far as personal health and safety are concerned, distinctions between the *Coccidioides* species are meaningless. They can all cause Valley Fever. Information in this book will benefit anyone concerned about any species or virulent strain of *Coccidioides.*

The main text of this book follows standardized capitalization and italicization rules for words such as coccidioidomycosis, *Coccidioides immitis (C. immitis)*, and *Coccidioides posadasii (C. posadasii)*. However, some quotations in this book are from medical journal articles that did not follow this formatting. The authors of this book left these unchanged to keep the quotations intact.

Endemic Area Maps and Information

Cocci can only be found in a few places in the world. These places where the fungus can grow are called "endemic areas." The principal endemic areas in the United States are Arizona (where 65% of America's infections are estimated to occur), and the desert valleys of California. In fact, Arizona[22] and Kern County in California (Bakersfield and surrounding areas) [128, 209, 210] have been called "hyperendemic" for this disease.

Other endemic areas in the United States are found in other parts of California, as well as in West Texas, New Mexico, Nevada, and Utah. The map on the following page shows shaded areas of the United States where mass testing revealed coccidioidomycosis as an endemic disease.

It is important to note that:

A) Two thirds of all Valley Fever cases are contracted in Arizona, with Phoenix and Tucson as the two most affected cities.

B) Kern County (Bakersfield) is the major endemic area in California.

C) There are also endemic areas in Mexico, Central America, and South America.

D) Environmental conditions have been known to blow spores hundreds of miles out of their original endemic areas to cause infections.

E) The mass testing that enabled these maps to be produced has not been repeated for half a century.

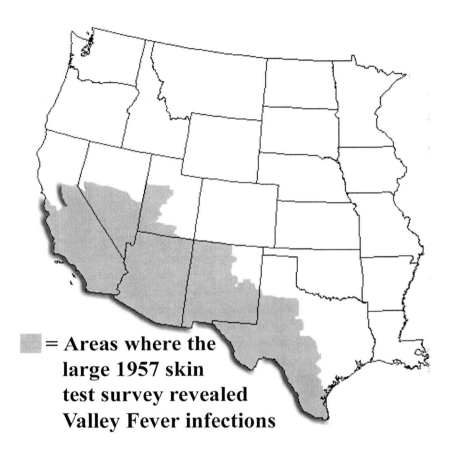

**= Areas where the
large 1957 skin
test survey revealed
Valley Fever infections**

    The next map shows areas the U.S. Geological Survey has
identified as endemic to the *Coccidioides* fungus. Notice the X at
the Dinosaur National Monument site in Utah, far to the north
of previously established endemic areas. All ten of the workers at
a DNM archeological site on June 19, 2001 became ill with Valley
Fever. The exact location of cocci's growth could not be
pinpointed for this particular outbreak, but it is suspected to
grow near the X.

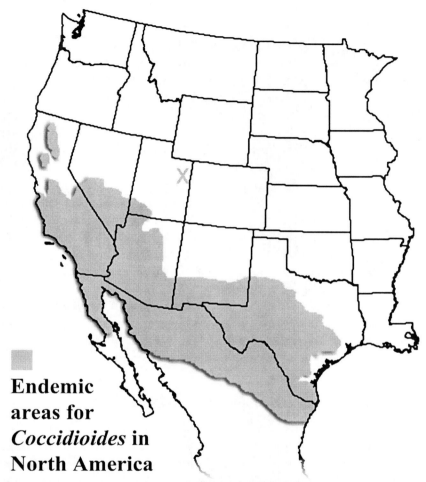

Endemic areas for *Coccidioides* in North America

These maps were created by Valley Fever Survivor™ based on source material from the U.S. Geological Survey and a publication by Edwards and Palmer.[77]

Internationally, the disease is known to infect people in northern Mexico (especially along the northwestern border with the United States), and parts of Central America and South America, although tracking of the disease in these countries is virtually non-existent.

The First Case

In 1891 an Argentinean soldier named Domingo Escurra was the first person diagnosed with coccidioidomycosis. After earning his degree, Buenos Aires medical student Alejandro Posadas studied Escurra's condition while working in the pathology lab of Robert Wernicke. This secured Posadas' place in Valley Fever history. Not only was coccidioidomycosis nicknamed Posadas-Wernicke Disease for a time, but the recently coined *posadasii* species of *Coccidioides* and the new drug posaconazole are both named in recognition of his work.

Escurra had been in good health before his onset of Valley Fever, but four years before visiting Posadas "he had noticed verrucous [wart-like] patches on his nose and right cheek, then on his thigh and back. At first no bigger than the head of a pin, the nodules enlarged, became ulcerated, and looked, Posadas said, very [much] like a cauliflower."[87]

Escurra's infection went into remission for a time, then relapsed until his "skin was everywhere covered by lesions" and massive dissemination attacked his internal organs. "In 1898, after seven years of recurrent fever and painful new eruptions, the patient finally died."[87]

The Ongoing Significance of Early Discoveries

Early in its study, *Coccidioides* spores were thought to resemble the protozoan parasite *Coccidia*, often found in chickens. To this day, the name of coccidioidomycosis still represents this early medical mistake. In addition, *Coccidioides* has nothing to do with streptococcal bacteria (also nicknamed "cocci"). Coccidioidomycosis also has many other nicknames such as "Desert Rheumatism," "Desert Fever," and "Arizona Flu" to name a few, but it is presently called "Valley Fever" most often.

By 1900, coccidioidomycosis was understood to be a fungal disease. After an outbreak in the 1930's in the San Joaquin Valley of California, this disease was given its nickname "San Joaquin Valley Fever," often shortened further to "Valley Fever."

The disease threatened national security during World War II when thousands of American soldiers became sickened while training in the Southwest. It even affects our military today, as seen during a 2002 Navy Seal training exercise in California when 45% of the squad fell ill with Valley Fever.[61]

> Information about veterans seeking a disability rating due to their Valley Fever will be included in an upcoming book. If you need the information right away for your own case, it is also available on this page at our web site: http://www.valleyfeversurvivor.com/vetinfo.html

Statistics and Comparisons

The 2007 statistics used are early numbers, and these often increase as the CDC or local health organizations are able to collate more data. 2006 data were still considered provisional in the January 4, 2008 issue of the CDC's Morbidity and Mortality Weekly Report.[41]

Arizona Statistics

1993	580
1994	578
1995	623
1996	655
1997	958
1998	1,474
1999	1,812
2000	1,917
2001	2,301
2002	3,118
2003	2,695
2004	3,665
2005	3,778
2006	5,535
2007	5,042

The table to the left shows the reported diagnoses of Valley Fever in the state of Arizona by year. Notice the increase of nearly ten times as many cases in 2006 compared to 1993, and that almost every year set a new record as Arizona's worst year for Valley Fever. Although 2007 had a slight drop instead of a rise in provisional cases, the provisionally reported numbers often rise when there is time for more complete data to come in. Therefore, the totals for 2007 may increase later. Laboratory reporting became required for Valley Fever in Arizona starting in 1997. The CDC has declared Valley Fever in Arizona an epidemic.

While the numbers to the left only indicate diagnoses reported to the state of Arizona, a CDC report[38] indicates that numbers might have been higher earlier— and it is not unusual for information from Arizona to conflict with information from the CDC, even though the CDC often obtains its information directly from Arizona's reports.

Hospital Cost Comparisons

In 1993, there were 659 coccidioidomycosis related hospital admissions, although reporting to the Arizona Department of Health Services ultimately only recorded 580 infections for that year. These admissions certainly included people who were infected before that year, repeat admissions among those who were diagnosed in 1993, and patients who were diagnosed in that year but did not have their infections reported. Direct costs in Arizona for all 659 coccidioidomycosis related hospital admissions totaled approximately $19 million.

Of those 659 patients:

66% had primary pulmonary cocci
20% had progressive cocci
6% had cocci meningitis
11% died overall
17% of patients aged 30-39 died, the highest fatality rate by age group.

It is now 2008, fifteen years later. Hospital costs have risen dramatically and so have the number of coccidioidomycosis infections. In 2005, the most recent year that data from the State Inpatient Database was available, there were 2,052 Valley Fever hospitalizations recorded in Arizona.[116] That number is more than triple the hospitalizations the CDC noted above.

If one were to estimate Valley Fever hospital costs based only on the increase in hospital admissions from 1993 to 2005, the bill would be over $59 million for 2005. The overall annual costs for Valley Fever are estimated to be 120 million dollars nationwide.[157]

In 1993 there were only 580 infections reported for the entire year. In 2007, the newly reported Valley Fever victims from a month and a half could easily eclipse that.

Also, over 29% of Arizona's hospitalized pneumonia cases are estimated to be misdiagnosed Valley Fever.[252] Based on the 2005 State Inpatient Database for Arizona, there were 45,899 hospitalized pneumonia cases (not including pneumonia known to be from Valley Fever).[116] If over 29% of these were truly undiagnosed Valley Fever, that means over 13,300 people were hospitalized but not diagnosed—and this is only an estimate of pneumonia, not any of the other clinical forms of coccidioidomycosis that can destroy someone's health.

California Statistics

Since California is ranked second as a major endemic state, the following chart features the five counties that reported the highest number of Valley Fever infections over a five year period:

County	2002	2003	2004	2005	2006
Kern	1,072	1,283	1,524	1,666	1,084*
Fresno	83	135	143	291	744*
Los Angeles	83	97	166	200	221*
Tulare	96	143	161	132	192*
Kings	50	42	83	52	192*
CA State Total	1,797	2,091	2,641	2,885	3,131

*The 2006 total was updated since the creation of this chart but updated county totals were not available by publication time

Since the total number of reported cases is estimated to be only 2% of the infections that occurred overall in California, the total for 2006 would be estimated at over **156,000** cocci infections. Notice that the state's total had nearly doubled, that Kings County's annual caseload increased by nearly **300%**, and that Fresno's annual caseload increased by nearly **800%** over this five year period.

Valley Fever vs. Tuberculosis

Tuberculosis (TB) made national headlines in 2007 with the quarantine of a suspected carrier of the drug resistant variety of *Mycobacterium tuberculosis*. We thought it would be worthwhile to show a comparison between TB and Valley Fever (VF).

This comparison clearly shows the seriousness of Valley Fever and the state and local governments' knowledge about it. It also sheds light on the lack of media attention and warnings about Valley Fever compared to other diseases like TB. These failings persist even with the increasing number of patients infected every year during this Valley Fever epidemic.

Valley Fever/Tuberculosis Comparison Chart

Facts about the diseases	TB	VF
It can mimic the symptoms of other diseases	Yes	Yes
Causes cough, fatigue, night sweats, fever and/or a variety of other symptoms	Yes	Yes
Can make people cough up blood	Yes	Yes
Potentially lethal	Yes	Yes
Can disseminate from the lungs to attack virtually any other organ	Yes	Yes
Can cause chronic symptoms	Yes	Yes
Can become dormant and then reactivate at any time, perhaps decades later, to sicken or kill its host	Yes	Yes
Can be resistant to drug treatment	Yes	Yes
Travelers can easily find information about how to avoid this disease	Yes	No
Commonly spread from person to person	Yes	No
Can be inhaled and contracted 365 days a year because it is a part of the air in the desert Southwest, especially Arizona and the San Joaquin Valley of California	No	Yes
The Centers for Disease Control (CDC) makes national and international pronouncements about its health risks	Yes	No
Repeatedly mentioned in national news stories as an important health topic	Yes	No
Regulated as a Select Agent for its potential use as a biological weapon in two federal antiterrorism laws	No	Yes
Germany invoked the Geneva Convention during World War II because it would be unacceptable for America to keep captured Nazis in Florence, AZ specifically because the prisoners caught this disease there. America agreed to move the prisoners.	No	Yes

Symptoms

Not every symptom below will necessarily occur in every case of Valley Fever. Every case can be different. Some patients experience many symptoms, some do not notice any symptoms (even if, for example, someone is not aware of a nodule growing in his or her lung), and some might have all of these symptoms.

Signs of Valley Fever

Below is a list of many possible Valley Fever (coccidioidomycosis) symptoms:

Flu-like symptoms	Malaise/chronic exhaustion
Fever	Muscle aches
Shortness of breath/wheezing	Muscle stiffness
Coughing (can be chronic and severe)	Joint pain
Coughing up blood	Joint swelling
Chest pain/pressure	Joint stiffness
Night sweats/Chills	Leg/ankle/foot swelling
Headaches	Photosensitivity
Nausea	*Vision problems/blindness
Loss of appetite	**Neck stiffness
Weight loss	**Inability to focus and concentrate
Rash	**Foot drop or partial paralysis
Burning sensations at various parts of the body (foot, joints, etc.)	**Severe head pain (as opposed to a normal headache)

*This can be a sign of lesions in the eye, but also a side effect of Vfend (voriconazole), a medication used to treat Valley Fever.
**These can be a sign of meningitis associated with Valley Fever and may, therefore, require aggressive antifungal therapy.

Valley Fever is often misdiagnosed as cancer, tuberculosis, or bacterial pneumonia. It can disseminate (spread) throughout the body. The fact that the symptoms of Valley Fever vary so greatly is a part of the reason misdiagnosis is so common. In addition, the lack of training and lack of accurate information available to doctors is a contributing factor in the frequent misdiagnoses of this devastating illness.

The disease can cause hydrocephalus (harmful pressure from spinal fluid on the brain), verrucose ulcers (wartlike outgrowths on the surface of organs and skin), arthralgias (joint pains), myalgias (muscle pains), otomycosis (fungal infection of the external ear canal), hypercalcemia (extra calcium in the blood that can be fatal) and other terrible conditions.

The simplest, fastest description of Valley Fever is that the disease can create lesions or inflammation in nearly any part of the body. Lytic lesions involve rupture of cell membranes, keratotic ulcers are scaly and wartlike, and the disease can create lesions on other internal organs or manifest in visible, hideous skin conditions.

Depending on where Valley Fever causes inflammation within the body, a patient may experience arthritis, conjunctivitis, endocarditis, meningitis, myocarditis, osteomyelitis, pleuritis, tenosynovitis, vasculitis or a variety of other painful or life-threatening conditions. Meningitis, the swelling of the brain's lining, is universally regarded as the most deadly and dangerous form of Valley Fever. It occurs frequently in patients who have the disease spread from their lung.

Valley Fever usually starts in the lungs and can disseminate to virtually any part of the body such as:

Skin	Lymph nodes
Bones	Eyes
Joints	Heart
Spine	Kidney
Brain	Thyroid
Liver	Uterus
Testicles	Genitourinary tract
Prostate	Gastrointestinal tract

Common and Undiagnosed Symptoms

The most common sites of Valley Fever's dissemination from the lungs are the skin, joints, bones, and meninges.[31] Perhaps because some parts of the body are routinely infected, some doctors do not routinely suspect other parts.

A Frightening Example

The prostate is commonly affected by Valley Fever, but not commonly recognized. Studies have shown that as many as 6% of autopsied Valley Fever patients have had the infection spread to the prostate, but by the time of an exhaustive 2004 medical review, only 13 cases could be found where patients with this symptom were actually diagnosed before they died.[248]

Doctors mention that an "antemortem diagnosis is rare" for prostate involvement in Valley Fever and this is an incredible understatement.[159] It is staggering to consider these 13 diagnoses compared to what 6% could represent from the millions of people who have been infected over the years. This incredible number of men were almost universally untreated, and because prostate and other genital lesions often have noticeable symptoms of discomfort, they almost universally suffered.[20]

Of the 13 cases diagnosed while the patients were still alive, very little information can be drawn for this symptom's specific risk factors. "The median age at the time of diagnosis of coccidioidomycosis prostatitis was 62 years (range, 44-72 years). Sixty-two percent of the patients were white, 15% were black, 15% were Hispanic, and 8% were Filipino."[248]

Why Valley Fever's Symptoms Make Diagnosis Difficult

With the potential to affect any or all areas of the body, Valley Fever can be profoundly different for each patient. At its simplest, most of Valley Fever's symptoms can be considered a matter of lesions or inflammation anywhere in the body.

When a lesion is visible on the skin, the problem might be more obvious than if the lesion were destroying part of the lung or a bone, but it can all be a part of the same disease. Likewise, inflamed fluid in the joints (rheumatoid arthritis) and inflamed lungs (pneumonia) may feel different, but they are common symptoms in Valley Fever.

Also, just as coccidioidomycosis became known as San Joaquin Valley Fever even though it can grow in areas far from the San Joaquin Valley, not every case has a fever. Many of Valley Fever's symptoms can occur due to many other diseases, and doctors commonly misdiagnose or treat it as those other diseases instead. This has prompted the following statement to be written in the New England Journal of Medicine:

> "The main difficulty in diagnosis is failure to consider coccidioidomycosis."[240]

Symptoms in Animals

The symptoms in this chapter also apply to Valley Fever in animals. The most common signs of veterinary Valley Fever are respiratory distress, coughing, fever, malaise, loss of appetite, lameness, and unexplained personality changes. These could be particularly significant if the animal was exposed to soil in an endemic area.

Please see our chapter titled "Valley Fever in Animals" for more information.

Risk Factors

Valley Fever is spread when soil in an endemic area with *Coccidioides* growth is disturbed. This has happened due to earthquakes, archeology, children digging in the sand, cars driving through an area, and even wind that blew spores 500 miles out of the endemic areas.[71] Anything that can disturb dust or soil can also release *Coccidioides* into the air. However, those who are closer to the soil disturbances may inhale many more spores, and consequently may increase the risk of a more severe infection.

Valley Fever at Work

"Although infection can result from ambient exposure within urban settings, persons involved in activities that disrupt *Coccidioides immitis*-contaminated soil (e.g., archaeologic excavations, construction, and military maneuvers) are more likely to become infected and to have increased morbidity."[239]

"Face masks should be used by persons in high-risk jobs in the endemic areas, such as agricultural workers, construction crews, telephone-post diggers, and archeologists."[23]

To make employers aware of the issues involved with bringing people into areas where they might contract Valley Fever, an article was written in the American Journal of Public Health in 1968. It stated that "the importation of any susceptible labor force into endemic areas carries with it the responsibility for reducing the rate and severity of infection through whatever dust control measures are possible and for providing a vigorous program of medical surveillance."[218]

Tourists are also unaware of the risk to their health, but the article was focused on occupational risk factors. Unfortunately, nearly half a century later, none of the medical surveillance and few dust control measures have become required for employees at risk.

Although dust control is an important element in the reduction of Valley Fever infections, it is often ignored or insufficient[257] in some work places. "Because soil disturbance (with the subsequent formation of dust) and extensive outdoor activity enhance the chances of infection with *C. immitis*, coccidioidomycosis can be considered an occupational hazard. Workers associated with agriculture (ranchers, farmers) or with other outdoor activities (construction workers, baseball players) are especially at risk of contracting the infection."[216]

The list of enhanced occupational risks can also include archeologists, anthropologists, gardeners, military personnel, anyone who comes near or disturbs bare soil that might contain this fungus, and anyone who works outdoors to breathe the natural air on a regular basis.

There is also an occupational risk for anyone who handles objects that may have been through endemic areas. Those at risk include mechanics,[211] "persons cleaning trucks that carried contaminated material"[216] museum workers,[219] and even those who fly on airplanes through endemic areas.[185]

> "Some individuals on two floors above a coccidioides laboratory were infected via a ventilation duct...In another instance, a movie director was infected during the filming of an artificially created dust storm with soil 'imported' from an area near Los Angeles to which *C. immitis* is endemic. It is likely that infections also result during the filming of dusty Western movies."[195]

Working in labs with Valley Fever can be a colossal risk unto itself, as the medical literature has shown. In the 1940's, Valley Fever infections were believed to have occurred in "most laboratories in which the organism has been studied."[232] Even recent 21st century medical literature reminds lab workers of the danger *Coccidioides* poses: "Laboratory samples are highly contagious and should be handled with care."[263] In fact, even those who are already infected and have an immune resistance face a severe risk of reactivation or reinfection due to "the massive type of exposure that can occur in a laboratory accident."[242]

As one might expect, with the need to train in desert environments and to have clear skies for flying, the military is also especially hard hit. There are currently 350,000 American military personnel in the areas endemic to Valley Fever, and many more who are sent through these bases either for training or as a brief stop before their next destinations.

> "Military physicians in particular must be vigilant for this disease, as there are large numbers of personnel stationed in the desert southwest and even more who pass through [bases in the endemic areas]. These personnel engage in activities and maneuvers that make them more susceptible to coccidioidomycosis."[105]

Even undertakers who are helping prepare those who are deceased from Valley Fever are not entirely safe. After an undertaker's unusual infection, a medical report suggested the following: "It may be appropriate to warn undertakers of the risk they incur in handling bodies of victims of disseminated coccidioidomycosis. The problem is not that of ordinary contagion, but of inoculation from a puncture wound."[129]

Valley Fever at Play

Whether traveling for business or pleasure, Valley Fever can be a major risk. Aside from the fact that the tiny spores can remain airborne for very long periods of time (and therefore be in the air when there does not appear to be any dust visible whatsoever), doctors state that "because the desert is inherently dusty, many cases of coccidioidomycosis are acquired just by driving through the disease-endemic area."[150]

Reports of children playing in their backyards[245] or in outdoor "mud forts"[208] have highlighted the enhanced risks of behavior that involves outdoor activities or time near the soil.

> Any time spent in the endemic areas can result in a Valley Fever infection because it only takes the inhalation of one spore to contract a potentially lethal infection.[94, 187, 227, 255]

> "The incidence of disease has been increasing with the expansion of city borders. Disease prevalence is now stretching across the globe due to rising tourist industries in endemic areas with high visitation rates by foreign travelers...First, the prevalence and distribution of coccidioidomycosis is increasing as is the likelihood of seeing its often unique and bizarre clinical manifestations and complications."[163]

Reports of Valley Fever appear to be associated with nearly any activity. People have been infected during high-risk events like off-road biking or exposure to a leaf blower's stirred-up air. They have also been infected while changing planes at the Phoenix airport, visiting health spas, or simply taking trips to the supermarket on clear days. "People who are having outdoor fun in endemic areas are at equal risk of exposure to *Coccidioides* as those who are at work in agricultural areas of Arizona and Southern California."[53]

Personal Risk Factors

Coccidioides is an equal opportunity biohazard so Valley Fever poses a danger to anyone who inhales a spore. However, the risk factors for the most severe, life-threatening conditions may worsen depending on circumstances that are specific to some patients. These risk factors often make dissemination (the spread of *Coccidioides* spores from the lung through the bloodstream) more likely. When Valley Fever disseminates, it can attack virtually any part of the body.

Mentioning these risk factors may save many lives, but their mere mention is a double edged sword.

For residents and tourists who don't want to think about the danger, it is wrong but easy to say "oh, I'm not in a high risk group so I don't have to worry about Valley Fever." The fact that Valley Fever has some very specific risk factors should never minimize the fact that any healthy person in any group can be infected and may suffer the most debilitating or deadly forms of the disease.

To date, thousands of people have contacted us at www.valleyfeversurvivor.com and few of the risk factors applied to the majority of people who contacted us. Further, recent data questions the importance of some historical risk factors and this is noted below where applicable. However, if you belong to a risk group and live in an endemic area, the following information may be vitally important.

"The desert Southwest attracts many visitors for business and pleasure. The increased mobility of Americans has widened the geographic impact of coccidioidal infection, making it a national problem. Moreover, the increase in nonwhite and immunosuppressed populations places a greater number of persons at high risk for developing disseminated coccidioidal infection. For all these reasons, it is important that physicians consider coccidioidomycosis in patients who traveled recently to states in which the organism is endemic. In addition, if organizations, whether military or civilian, that regularly send persons into coccidioides-endemic regions would inform these persons about the potential of infection, diagnosis of this mycosis outside *C. immitis*-endemic regions might be facilitated."[239]

Men at Risk

In most Valley Fever epidemics, men were reported to have dissemination more often than women.[177] The early 1990's outbreak in Kern County, California provided a striking example. Males had 76% of the disseminated infections while they represented only 52% of the population.[11]

Pregnancy

While men ordinarily tend to have a higher risk for severe Valley Fever than women, the risk for women becomes even higher during pregnancy. Disseminated Valley Fever occurs up to 100 times as often in pregnant women than in the general population.[68] Another study shows pregnant women were ten times more likely to suffer the most severe Valley Fever symptoms than non-pregnant women who also had the disease.[35]

While dissemination from the lung is important, the lung infection itself can also be devastating. It is well known that pneumonia can cause a "systemic toxicity" in the mother, which "includes electrolyte imbalance, dehydration, and acidosis. These in turn result in a high incidence of abortion, premature birth, and fetal death in utero." Perhaps that is why "the main complication of this disorder during the first trimester of pregnancy was a tendency to abort" rather than to kill the mother outright as it does more often in the third trimester of pregnancy.[162]

"The potential for devastating illness is well documented" because pregnancy causes a variety of hormonal and immune system changes that put the mother at risk. It is even possible for the fetus to be at risk, either from the death of the mother, "therapeutic abortion," or by spread of *Coccidioides* through the placenta.[237] While the placenta can normally filter the spores, this protection is not absolute.[165] Of course, it is also possible, if the child is born in an endemic area, that its nursery or other area could have air that would provide a deadly dose of Valley Fever as well.[230]

Since even the milder drugs that fight Valley Fever can cause birth defects, pregnant women in need of antifungal medication for their Valley Fever must be given amphotericin B.[141] This drug is infamously harsh and described in our Drugs and Treatment Chapter.

> "The high risk of maternal death and fetal wastage in disseminated coccidioidomycosis compels aggressive management."[174]

Race

For decades, *Coccidioides* has been evaluated as a race-specific weapon of biological warfare.[179] Even with the enhanced risks involved in pregnancy for all races, pregnant black women are 13 times more likely to suffer disseminated Valley Fever than pregnant Caucasians.[60]

Hispanics, Asians, and Native Americans are often considered to suffer from Valley Fever with the worst symptoms more often than Caucasians.[48, 79, 177, 210] People of Filipino and black heritage, however, are widely known to have the most severe cases more often than other races. The risk is so high, in fact, that a 1958 textbook made the following off-handed statement for the benefit of black and Filipino lab workers:

> "Handling *Coccidioides immitis* without proper [laboratory] precautions is foolhardy—and for members of certain races may be suicidal."[86]

The reasons are clear and just as valid today. Doctors have stated that "Filipinos and African Americans have been shown to have up to a 200-fold increased risk of disseminated disease and an increased mortality rate"[62] or noted the "much greater mortality rate in dark-skinned people (Mexicans, Filipinos, and Blacks). They are 25 times more likely to develop progressive disease and death."[71]

The upper end of the numbers for the likelihood of dissemination and death for Filipinos with Valley Fever probably came from a classic study[106] in Kern County from 1901-1936. This study noted a 19,118% greater chance of death for Filipinos with Valley Fever than Caucasians. This study also found African Americans were 2,236% more likely to die of their Valley Fever cases than Caucasians. Native Americans were 861% more likely to die. Persons of Mexican and Japanese descent were both listed as being about 400% more likely to die than Caucasians.

The study also showed that persons of Chinese descent frequently died from Valley Fever with rates 2,661% above the Caucasian death rate. This statistic has not been seen in later literature, perhaps because there were few other subdivided Asian studies outside the Filipino ethnicity to make further judgments in the earlier surveys.[89] Also, "Asian" has since been used as a generalized statistical group when studying cocci risk factors, although Filipinos are often evaluated separately in statistics due to their dramatically increased risk.

Some of the estimates above were reduced by roughly 75% in 1970's surveys due to differences in living conditions and sample sizes, but the racial risks remain high at any time.[143]

In other early surveys, it appeared that many "autopsies were not done with the enthusiastic thoroughness" needed to check whether meningitis from Valley Fever had caused some deaths in any racial group and might have added further to the toll.[128] In later surveys the recorded risks had been increased beyond all original suspicions. For example, in 1999 the rate of dissemination in African Americans was estimated at 28 times the Caucasian rate.[168]

At different times and locations the studies have ranges of estimates that are obviously large, but an important fact remains: Some non-Caucasian groups are at a dramatically greater risk of severe Valley Fever. Also, regardless of other variations in the risk categories, when adjusted by race Filipinos are universally considered first and African Americans are usually second in the rates of dissemination. This is true in old[106] and new[30] outbreaks alike. These groups are typically considered to have their Valley Fever disseminate "20 to 30 times as often" as Caucasians.[259] Numbers have been even higher in other reports.[59]

Aside from the threat of dissemination itself, there are other race-specific issues, like the likelihood of bone and joint involvement. Although African Americans are minorities in the endemic areas, they represented 47% of the positive cases in one study.[134] Another study found African Americans to have 51% of bone and joint dissemination cases overall.[221] In a review of 409 people infected with Valley Fever, 18% were found to have chronic suffering from the disease. "The chronic syndrome, characterized by a prolonged course sometimes lasting up to 30 years, is more common in pigmented races than in whites."[138]

Of course, even though it has been said that pigmentation or "dark skin" is a risk factor,[90, 138] the risk of this disease is less a matter of skin color and more a matter of other attributes.[128] These attributes may be blood type factors,[168] differences in histocompatibility complex genes (which control the immune response),[210] or other unknown factors.[71] Sometimes a genetic factor that leaves one race more susceptible to severe Valley Fever may not do the same to a person of another race.[168]

Even with the information of the high incidence in Filipinos, African Americans have also borne a risk of severe Valley Fever. Coccidioidomycosis can be so harmful to black patients that doctors in one study "did not find a higher rate of reported disseminated coccidioidomycosis in black persons with AIDS. Black race may not be associated with an increased risk for disseminated coccidioidomycosis among persons with AIDS because immunosuppression by HIV among nonblack persons may make them as susceptible to dissemination."[145]

> The doctors here essentially said that, as far as Valley Fever is concerned, being black may be just as dangerous as having AIDS.

Everyone is aware of the way AIDS can destroy a person's health and a person's life. By contrast, few people are aware of Valley Fever, even though their race might put them at equal risk of severe illness from it as AIDS patients. This is something every person who visits, passes through, or lives in the Southwest must consider.

Since this disease can obviously be debilitating and easy to contract in endemic areas, race-based suggestions have been made about employment in high-risk jobs like soil moving and construction. One recommendation said that unless black and Filipino workers had already been infected (thereby having an immune resistance to light *Coccidioides* exposures) "they should whenever possible be assigned to work in areas or at jobs where exposure to high concentrations of spores will be minimal."[218]

Although this suggestion is essentially racial discrimination in the workplace, it was not made because of hateful prejudice but respect for life. No information could be found to indicate whether this potentially life-saving suggestion has ever been instituted.

Ironically, for all the race-based risk factors, Caucasians are almost always the most affected by Valley Fever—Even in the classic study[106] that first demonstrated dramatically higher death rates in other groups, the actual number of whites that died of Valley Fever was higher than any other race. This is simply because the majority of the area's population was white. As racial diversity increases in the Southwest, it may be reasonable to expect a corresponding increase in the overall severity and death toll of the Valley Fever epidemic.

Age

Valley Fever may affect the elderly and children with far more debilitating cases.[79, 153]

Often "the association of age with mortality tends to be understated."[10]

A CDC report said that patients over 65 years of age in Arizona are more than five times as likely to be diagnosed with this disease as patients in the 15-24 year-old group. The report also showed that 65+ seniors have twice the diagnosis rate of the 25-34 and 35-44 year-old age groups. Suggested possibilities for the more frequent diagnoses were increased likelihood to seek medical attention or the chronic infections that tend to be more frequent in seniors.[38]

A 2001 study of an outbreak in Kern County, California also highlights the enhanced risk of severe Valley Fever in elderly patients.[210] The physiological conditions of advanced age are suggested to be responsible for the increased risk, whether in travelers or lifelong residents.[160]

Valley Fever is also common in the very young.[158] Meningitis and other forms of dissemination were even more common in children than adults in a study in Mexico. This study also reported the occurrence of "epidemics of infantile coccidioidomycosis."[33] An American retrospective report found that nationwide Valley Fever hospitalizations in children during 2002 led to an 8.5% death rate, which was higher than the 5.7% adult death rate.[49] A lack of scientific research could contribute to this problem. "Studies abound on the disease in adults, but studies addressing dissemination in the child pale in comparison."[149]

The enhanced risk for severe disease still cannot be generalized to all circumstances. A study in California showed children under the age of five to be the least likely age group to be infected.[210] Also, although it did not rate severity, it is interesting to note that 2006 case reporting in Los Angeles County has shown that infections were most frequently reported in the group aged 15-35 years old,[166] not children or the elderly.

Since all ages are at risk, it may take increased active surveillance of the disease before all age-based risk factors can be confirmed.

Immune System Health

There are many ways for an immune system to become compromised, leading to a severe Valley Fever infection or a reactivation of a previous, possibly dormant infection. "Reactivation has been described in pregnant women, patients with human immunodeficiency virus, [organ] transplant patients treated with immunosuppressive agents [for their organ graft] and even in apparently healthy individuals."[266] Even diabetes and malnutrition are risk factors. Since the immune system's white blood cells fight the rapidly multiplying *Coccidioides* parasitic cells to keep them in check, a damaged immune system can make a case of Valley Fever much worse.[31, 194, 254, 258]

"From the beginning of the AIDS epidemic in 1981 to June 1989" cases of disseminated Valley Fever "accounted for 6% of all cases of AIDS reported" to the State of Arizona.[91]

Cases in other groups with immune disorders are also higher. The fact that most Valley Fever lab tests check for antibodies poses another problem: An immunocompromised condition can reduce the production of antibodies, so people who might ordinarily test positive for the disease could falsely test negative instead.[7]

> "Despite antifungal therapy" in a study of AIDS patients, a full quarter of the patients "died within 90 days of the diagnosis of coccidioidomycosis." Considering what a problem diagnosis can be and how many people must have been undiagnosed, AIDS patients still had a rate of diagnosis 6,711 times the rate in the general population, underscoring the severity.[261]

However, this risk should not be overstated to the general population because virtually any disease is worse when the immune system is not functioning normally. "Mortality rates are 40 to 60 percent for patients without concomitant HIV infection" in Valley Fever patients with meningitis.[148] This complication is clearly serious even for patients who do not have HIV/AIDS. In a study of Valley Fever pneumonia autopsies from the San Joaquin Valley, 98% of the victims did not have an immunocompromised condition. The conclusion is clear: "Fatal coccidioidal pneumonia is certainly not confined to the immunocompromised host."[242]

Before the increased use of immunosuppressive drug therapy and the appearance of HIV/AIDS, only 2% of Valley Fever cases had an underlying illness. *Coccidioides* clearly threatens public health regardless of any individual's immune status.[24] A study of recent hospitalization data found that only 12% of hospitalized Valley Fever patients had an underlying immunocompromising condition.[49] From our own questionnaires at www.valleyfeversurvivor.com to date, the vast majority of people apparently had healthy immune systems when they had contracted Valley Fever.

The key point to remember about this risk factor is that everyone is just as likely to contract Valley Fever. However, people with weakened immune systems are dramatically more likely to suffer chronic, severe, and lethal Valley Fever once they do contract it.

Smoking

> "Smoking was found to be the most important preventable cause of acute symptomatic coccidioidomycosis in this population, independent of duration of Arizona residence, underlying illnesses, or other factors. The [statistical risk calculation] suggests that about one-half of all cases of acute coccidioidomycosis would not have occurred in the absence of cigarette smoking. Other studies have also recently linked smoking with increased susceptibility to bacterial and mycotic pathogens acquired via the respiratory route."[160]

Smoking has repeatedly been correlated with patients who have severe Valley Fever cases. [11, 70, 73, 160]

A correlation is not conclusive, but certainly a worthwhile consideration for any disease that starts in the lung. If it isn't bad enough that Valley Fever causes destruction or inflammation anywhere in the body, it can also be misdiagnosed as lung cancer, which in turn can lead to even more destruction if lesions are removed that may not have needed removal.[107] Doctors might easily believe that a history of smoking led to the lesion when it may actually be due to Valley Fever.

Alcohol

Alcohol use has been believed to affect Valley Fever[212, 258] and serious alcohol consumption has been associated with more severe Valley Fever in some patients.[11] There is room for disagreement on this point since some doctors' studies had too few people involved "to form strong conclusions" on the topic.[22] Moreover, some other articles did not specifically find a direct link between severity of this disease and alcohol consumption.[105, 210]

Corticosteroids and Hormones

> "Under no circumstances should adrenal steroids or cortisone preparations be used, as these may cause rapid dissemination of a focalizing primary infection."[259]

Doctors have found a handful of specific uses for corticosteroids in Valley Fever since the above quotation's first

printing. For example, in a patient with Valley Fever that led to Acute Respiratory Distress Syndrome and a rib lesion, doctors carefully combined antifungal drugs with corticosteroids.[223] However, corticosteroids can harm the immune system in ways that enable some of Valley Fever's worst complications to arise.
[105, 110, 114, 121, 144, 231, 240, 266]

Studies show that the growth and maturation of *Coccidioides* spp. is stimulated by human sex hormones such as testosterone and progesterone. This may be why some treatments have caused many cocci cases to worsen.[105, 144, 240] Increased hormone levels play a role in the increased danger to pregnant women with Valley Fever,[123] but other uses of hormones (for example, hormone replacement therapy) have not been studied with this disease.

Other Drugs

Even taking antibiotics for bacterial infections may cause problems or work in combination with antifungal treatment to make Valley Fever more severe.[78, 132] Since a lack of soil competition from other bacteria and fungi appears to allow *Coccidioides* to grow better in the soil[152] and during in vitro studies,[131] perhaps this same effect occurs in the body as well.

Valley Fever can cause arthritis, so the following information about the arthritis drug Remicade (infliximab) is important. In the ATTRACT international drug studies, Remicade was linked to five deaths: "...one died of pulmonary embolism, two died of cardiopulmonary events, one died of tuberculosis and one died of coccidioidomycosis ('Valley Fever')."[74] This drug is known to cause nervous system disorders and weaken the immune system, increasing the likelihood of the most severe complications of opportunistic infections such as tuberculosis and Valley Fever.

Other reported side effects include the activation of septic arthritis, multiple sclerosis, cancer, congestive heart failure, and more.[74] We encourage Valley Fever patients who use or are considering using Remicade to discuss this with their physician. Ironically, some legal complaints against the pharmaceutical company read very much like a list of complaints that could be made against Valley Fever's endemic states.[207]

Perhaps other drugs could also cause significant side effects in Valley Fever patients, but a comprehensive list is not available.

Blood Type

One study of Valley Fever patients found that blood type B or AB was associated with 41.7% of patients with dissemination[52] and this appears to agree with other statements of higher risk in those with blood type B.[168, 262]

Organ Transplants

Like the West Nile Virus, Valley Fever has been transferred from organ donors to recipients.[18, 21, 180, 247, 262]

Increased testing and improved record keeping of organ donors' medical histories are essential. Also, many transplant recipients require immunosuppressive drugs that dramatically increase the risk of severe Valley Fever.

Blood Transfusions: A Risk Factor?

Since disseminated coccidioidal infections spread through the bloodstream, sometimes without patients feeling the effects of the disease, it seems intuitive that blood transfusions might be able to spread the disease. However, the American Association of Blood Banks does not check the blood supply for *Coccidioides*. We sincerely hope this will change, as it is untested as to whether a person could be infected by a blood transfusion.[65]

Poverty

Even the risk of "socioeconomic status" with an annual income below $15,000 was seen to be a risk factor for the most serious Valley Fever conditions.[210] This finding may be due to any number of reasons, from increased likelihood to work in dusty environments where high doses of spores could be inhaled, to a lack of ability to pay for medical care and thus only visiting doctors when symptoms are at their worst.

Frequently Asked Questions

In the years since we established
www.valleyfeversurvivor.com we have received many similar
questions over and over. It makes sense for us to use a
Frequently Asked Question format so readers can have all the
information they want quickly.

What is Valley Fever?
Valley Fever is the common name for the parasitic fungal
disease coccidioidomycosis. Recent statistics show that Valley
Fever causes symptoms in over half of the people who are
infected.[54]

Nearly half will not feel sick immediately upon infection,
but most will have symptoms including fever, rashes, headaches,
severe abscesses and lesions in nearly any part of the body.
Valley Fever can even kill its victims through pneumonia,
meningitis, and other horrors in its worst cases, or activate
decades after the initial infection. Please see our Symptoms
Chapter.

Who can contract Valley Fever?
Any person, any mammal, and some other animals can
contract Valley Fever, regardless of age or health. It has been an
epidemic in humans for years. All it takes is inhaling one spore.

How can I contract Valley Fever?
Infection is caused by inhaling the fungal spores of
Coccidioides spp. (*C. immitis* or *C. posadasii*). All anyone has to do is
take a breath where these spores are airborne. The spores are
approximately the same size as anthrax spores and the wind can
carry them up to 500 miles from their source.[71]

The spores can come through ventilation systems or can
be inhaled outdoors whether in the city, country, or desert
environment of an endemic region. These spores become
parasites in your lung and can spread through the bloodstream.

From there they can go virtually anywhere in the body. This spread from the lung is called dissemination.

An infection can also be caused if *Coccidioides* spores enter an open cut or wound. This is known as a cutaneous infection, but is far less common than when spores are inhaled.

Is Valley Fever contagious from person to person, animal to person, or person to animal?

It is not contagious like the common cold. However, infectious spores have been passed cutaneously between open wounds. This is a rare event that happens most often to medical professionals, people handling deceased contaminated animals, or those handling needles with infectious *Coccidioides* spores.

The disease has also been passed from donated organs to organ recipients, resulting in death in some cases. Although some donated organs are checked for Valley Fever, mistakes can be deadly—especially considering that all organ transplant patients are already at a greater risk for dissemination if infected because of the immune deficiencies caused by the transplant process.

We are also unsure about the safety of the blood supply. Valley Fever disseminates through the bloodstream to other parts of the body, and people who donate blood may not be aware of the fungal spherules or endospores in their blood at the time. It is not known whether donated blood with *Coccidioides* in it can infect the recipient. We have not been able to locate any research to confirm or deny this possibility and the American Association of Blood Banks admits they do not test for this disease.

In summary, there are four confirmed ways to be infected and an unconfirmed fifth possibility:

1.   Inhalation of spores from the air into the lung. Most Valley Fever cases are contracted this way.
2.   Open lesions or cuts that come into contact with *Coccidioides* spores.
3.   Receiving a Valley Fever infected organ during an organ transplant.
4.   Accidental infection when people working with live spores have injected themselves with *Coccidioides*. This

usually occurs with scientists, but has even happened to a mortician who prepared a Valley Fever victim's body.

5. Since the CDC to date has ignored our request to screen the blood supply for Valley Fever and the disease disseminates through the bloodstream, there is no way to be certain whether it could be transmitted through a blood transfusion. This is a reasonable possibility to consider because parasitic *Coccidioides* endospores are smaller than red blood cells. The CDC had previously been wrong about the possibility of infection from other blood borne illnesses such as the West Nile Virus.

Is there a cure for Valley Fever?

No. Once a person or animal has contracted Valley Fever, the infection remains for life. Even if you were infected but lucky enough for your infection to become dormant, there is a risk that the disease can activate or reactivate at any time in your life to require surgeries, cause chronic illness, and possibly result in death. Nikkomycin Z is a potential cure that has been known for decades but only recently has been given proper funding for study. It is described further in our Drugs and Treatment Chapter.

Is there a vaccine for Valley Fever?

For many years the Valley Fever Vaccine Project in California and Dr. Garry Cole at the University of Texas at San Antonio (UTSA) each have been working on vaccines. However, they are facing budgetary difficulties. Please read Appendix A: Organizations and Internet Resources to find out more about them and how to donate to them.

Is Valley Fever more common in some endemic states than others?

Yes. Historically, Arizona has had 65% of America's diagnosed Valley Fever cases, primarily in Maricopa and Pima Counties (Phoenix and Tucson), where the bulk of Arizona's population lives. Infection rates are also particularly high in Kern County and other parts of California. Bakersfield has been considered "hyperendemic." Coccidioidomycosis was nicknamed

"San Joaquin Valley Fever" because California's San Joaquin Valley is considered highly endemic.

How can I find a doctor in my area that knows about Valley Fever?

There was a time when you could contact the Valley Fever Center for Excellence to get recommendations for doctors. Unfortunately in 2004 they had informed us this is no longer the case. The best we can suggest is that you should interview pulmonologists and infectious disease doctors in your local area and ask them how many people with coccidioidomycosis they have treated successfully. Infectious disease doctors are often more aware of the disease than general practitioners and pulmonologists, but many still cling to misconceptions about the disease. Please share the information in this book with your medical practitioners. In addition, you can recommend that your doctor read the information at www.valleyfeversurvivor.com to have the most accurate, up-to-date information on this disease.

If your doctor refuses to listen to you or to look at new information, we suggest you consider finding another physician. A doctor's ego is not as important as your health. Also, when searching for new doctors, be sure to ask the staff any questions you may have. If you find that they are rude or uncooperative, remember that the staff's attitude is often a reflection of the doctor's behavior.

Are doctors in endemic areas (Arizona and California, especially) likely to take Valley Fever more seriously than out-of-state doctors?

A doctor's location does not appear to be important. Many doctors who practice in the most heavily endemic areas have shown themselves to be dangerously ignorant or incompetent when it comes to this disease. Most doctors outside the endemic areas are not considered likely to know about the disease in-depth, but some do.

Some of our questionnaire respondents reported that knowledgeable doctors who had visited their hospital corrected their local doctor's misdiagnosis and mistreatment, even though the visiting doctor was not from an area endemic to Valley Fever.

Obviously a local doctor should be fully aware of local endemic diseases, but the experience of many patients suggests that this is not the case. The chapter titled "What You Need to Know Before You See A Doctor" may provide tips to help you find a doctor that is knowledgeable about Valley Fever.

What can a doctor do to test for Valley Fever?

This question is extensively covered in our Testing and Diagnosis Chapter.

My doctor wants me to take antifungal drugs. How long will I need to be on the medication? Do my symptoms have to be serious?

Some Valley Fever patients may require lifelong antifungal treatment. This may be true in some people even if their symptoms do not appear to be terrible. If you continue to run a titer your physician will probably want you to stay on antifungals because ongoing positive titer tests often suggest Valley Fever is still active in your body.

My Valley Fever has been misdiagnosed as cancer. Does this happen very often?

Yes. Lung lesions are often misdiagnosed as cancer, surgically cut out of the lung, and then diagnosed as Valley Fever after the fact. This causes a great deal of unnecessary pain to the patient's body and stress in personal relationships. We recommend that you ask your doctor if a fine needle lung nodule biopsy could be performed instead of starting with major surgery. This may save part of your lung if you have been in, passed through, or received packages from an endemic region, as the suspected cancer may actually be a Valley Fever infection.

I live in an endemic zone and was told Valley Fever was a benign disease. Is that true?

It can make you sick, cause fungal abscesses or lesions, debilitate you, cripple you for life, or kill you. It can be unbearably painful and is definitely not a benign disease. The misconception that Valley Fever is benign was started because of a medical focus on the common flu-like symptoms that start many Valley Fever cases, and also the potential for an immune resistance, which is explained later in this chapter.

I have cats, dogs, horses and/or other animals. Are they safe from Valley Fever?

All mammals (including cats, dogs, horses, dolphins, etc.) and some other animals are susceptible to the disease. It is considered an epidemic in dogs. There have been no confirmed cases in birds to date.

Did I contract Valley Fever because I have another disease?

No. People contract the disease simply by inhaling a *Coccidioides* sp. spore. Some diseases are more likely to allow a Valley Fever case to be more severe, but everyone can contract Valley Fever because everyone needs to breathe.

Who is at the greatest risk for the worst Valley Fever infections?

Senior citizens and young children under five years old, people with immune disorders like HIV/AIDS, organ transplant recipients, diabetics, pregnant women, and some races (particularly blacks and Filipinos) have historically been known to have the worst cases. People working close to the soil (construction workers, gardeners, etc.) are also at a higher risk than the general population because they are likely to inhale many more spores of the fungus as the spores are being stirred up.

However, it is important to repeat that ANYONE can have a severe or fatal infection no matter how healthy they are and even if they don't have any risk factors. For example, a 2006 article in Clinical Infectious Diseases reviewed hospital data to show that 86.3% of child patients and 87.5% of adult patients hospitalized with Valley Fever had healthy immune systems.[49]

If I have an immune deficiency, are my chances of contracting Valley Fever any greater?

Anyone in an endemic area has an equal chance to inhale the fungal spores, but with an immune deficiency chances of having a *severe* case of the disease are much greater. There is a significant risk for the most severe Valley Fever cases in people who go to an endemic area while their immune systems are severely weakened.

When AIDS and VF were being recognized as a serious combination in patients, a study showed that 60% of these patients died, even though most had antifungal treatment. Of those who died, 68% died in a median 54 days.[229] Another study showed a 42% death rate over seven years.[91] A more recent study of VF patients with AIDS said a quarter of the patients "died within 90 days of the diagnosis of coccidioidomycosis."[261]

Since I don't have an immune deficiency, I don't have to worry about Valley Fever, right?

No. As in the previous question, it changes the odds of dissemination but it doesn't mean you won't contract the disease or have a severe case. Your odds of contracting the disease do not change whether or not you have an immune deficiency since this parasitic fungal infection is acquired simply by breathing. More healthy people contract Valley Fever than immunocompromised people. Further, even if someone doesn't have an immune deficiency now, that doesn't guarantee his or her health for a lifetime—AIDS, organ transplantation, cancer treatments, and many other drugs are known to reduce immune effectiveness, potentially allowing for a fresh reactivation of the host's dormant Valley Fever.

I already have Valley Fever. Do I have a lifetime immunity to the disease?

Once a person is infected with Valley Fever an *immune resistance* takes effect in the body, but this does not mean total immunity in the sense that a person could never suffer from the disease again. This resistance is far from a guarantee of safety.

There are no major long term studies specifically following people with dormant Valley Fever to observe how they are struck by it later in life. However, there are plenty of studies and medical reviews following patients who relapsed severely after seemingly defeating the disease with medication. Documentation has also proven that patients' infections relapsed (or activated for the first time) years after leaving the endemic zones where they could have contracted Valley Fever.[9, 20, 36, 54 63, 142, 190]

It is therefore impossible for any medical professional to say that people and animals cannot be reinfected. In fact, there are many cases of animal testing and even laboratory personnel with dormant Valley Fever who accidentally inhaled large doses of spores in the lab. They subsequently had new infections that overcame their immune resistance, proving reinfection is possible.[214, 227]

Fifteen trillion *Coccidioides* arthroconidia can fit into a cubic inch.[167, 253] It is impossible to predict when any breath of air in Arizona or another endemic area might contain enough spores to demolish an infected person's immune resistance.

With laboratory infections excluded, there is presently only one way to tell the difference between a reactivation and an infection caused by the inhalation of more spores: That is when the patient has positive cultures of two or more lesions and testing proves that at least one lesion was caused by a different strain of *Coccidioides* than another lesion.

I'm pregnant. Does this matter for my Valley Fever case?

Valley Fever can strike pregnant women with much more severe cases than non-pregnant women, particularly in the third trimester. Many antifungal drugs can cause birth defects to a developing fetus and patients may be put on these drugs for life. Doctors have recommended that some of these women should never have children. This can be devastating to young girls who wanted to become mothers one day.

Is there a greater risk of Valley Fever at certain times of the year?

Valley Fever can be contracted all year round, but higher infection rates occur at certain times of the year. In Arizona the largest outbreaks are usually from June through July and October through November.[57] In California, the usual outbreaks are from June through November.[100]

Will a bandana or dust mask protect me from contracting Valley Fever if it is dusty outside?

No. Since the spores that cause Valley Fever are so minute (approximately the same size as the anthrax spore), ordinary dust masks and bandanas cannot prevent you from being infected. The microscopic spores can pass through the mask like marbles dropped through a fishing net.

A respirator that prevents the inhalation of particles 2-4 micrometers in size may help. Ordinary N95 or N100 respirators are often sold as paper masks and will almost certainly let spores through the sides since they can't form a perfect seal around the face. Miner's masks (or other masks with a complete seal and protection against 2-4 micrometer particles) can provide the needed protection. Also, facial hair prevents the seal that is necessary for the effectiveness of many masks.

What can I do to protect myself from Valley Fever?

Avoid going to any endemic region. However, if you live in or visit an endemic area to *Coccidioides*, it is helpful to keep car vents closed, avoid going out during dust storms, and avoid being near or participating in soil-disturbing activities (gardening, digging, etc). Visible dust does not need to be in the air for *Coccidioides* spores to be present. Even these measures may not keep you completely safe, but they are important precautions. The masks described above may also help.

I heard of someone who contracted Valley Fever but never went to an endemic area. How is this possible?

Sometimes fungi like *C. immitis* and *C. posadasii* can rest on inanimate objects like clothing, pottery, blankets, packing material, construction equipment, or even in the soil of potted plants, etc. and these products could be shipped elsewhere with the biohazard intact. This might be more likely on dusty objects or objects purchased outdoors at roadside stands in an endemic region. The items that had the spores on them are referred to as *fomites*. This book's introduction provides examples of fomite transmission.

If I live in a non-endemic area (where *Coccidioides sp.* does not grow), does that mean I'm safe?

If you remain more than 500 miles away from any known endemic area, the answer may be yes. Winds have only been known to spread the spores up to 500 miles. However, some focal endemic areas have been discovered far from the expected areas, like the Dinosaur National Monument outbreak in northern Utah in June 2001.

Is it possible to pass through an endemic state for only a short time and still contract Valley Fever?

Yes. One person was in Phoenix only to change planes at the airport and contracted a Valley Fever infection at that time.[27] People have also contracted Valley Fever while just driving through endemic states.

Is it safe to come to an endemic state for just a short stay such as a baseball game, the Fiesta Bowl, the Tucson Gem and Jewelry show, etc?

No. There is always a risk of contracting Valley Fever. Although there are specific risk factors, anyone can contract Valley Fever at any time. All you need to do is inhale one microscopic spore of the airborne fungal parasite.

I have shunt tubing and I'm infected with Valley Fever. My Valley Fever case appeared to be better for a while but suddenly got worse. Is this a normal reactivation of my infection?

It may not be. In some Valley Fever cases, shunt tubing can grow a biofilm that resists antifungal treatment. You may wish to share a medical journal article titled "Biofilm on Ventriculo-Peritoneal Shunt Tubing as a Cause of Treatment Failure in Coccidioidal Meningitis"[66] with your doctor if you have shunt tubing and a Valley Fever infection. A web link to this article is included below for your use:

http://www.cdc.gov/ncidod/eid/vol8no4/01-0103.htm

Do the state governments where Valley Fever is contracted know about this disease?

Yes. The endemic states' legislators all know about this disease and the Valley Fever Center for Excellence has sent information to all United States Senators as well.

What are the endemic states doing to fund research?

Arizona does not fund any Valley Fever organization directly. For over a decade, almost every year has produced what was considered Arizona's worst Valley Fever outbreak in recorded history, only to be outdone again by the following year. Ultimately with the colossal outbreak in 2006, $50,000 in emergency funds were spent to train Arizona's doctors to recognize Valley Fever. No funding for Valley Fever medical research has yet been appropriated by the state.

California had been funding the Valley Fever Americas Foundation's vaccine project but cut the funding by nearly one and a half million dollars due to statewide budgetary problems. Some of its funding has since been continued, but full funding is not a sure thing to the vaccine's successful completion. In Appendix A: Organizations and Internet Resources we show how you can donate to this very important organization.

I thought a warm, dry, sunny climate like Arizona and Southern California was good for my health. That's what my doctor tells me. Why should I believe otherwise?

Some people will certainly enjoy the warmth, the dryness, and the sun. It's just the incurable, debilitating, painful, and potentially fatal *Coccidioides spp.* fungal parasites that we seek to warn people about. Since everyone has to breathe and that is mainly how Valley Fever is contracted in these endemic regions, you must be aware of this to decide whether the climate matters more than the health risk.

I know someone who died from Valley Fever. If I contract it, does that mean I will die too?

Every case can be different. Remember that Valley Fever may not cause any problems initially and some cases resolve without the need for medication. Obtaining prompt medical care and early diagnosis may prevent dissemination and some of Valley Fever's worst health problems.

My titers have recently become lower, but my Valley Fever symptoms feel worse. How is this possible and what could this mean?

A lower number on the Valley Fever complement fixation titer is usually associated with an improvement of the patient's symptoms, but this link is not absolute. This is because the titer tests are for antibodies against Valley Fever, and while antibodies are useful in blood tests for doctors' diagnoses, they are not effective when fighting the disease. It is cell-mediated immunity that fights Valley Fever, specifically with white blood cells called T lymphocytes.[127]

A decreased antibody response could be due to...

A) an immune system problem,
B) the fact that a decrease in antibody response doesn't necessarily have anything to do with the course of the disease (Valley Fever may actually be getting worse), or
C) a medical error during testing or transportation of test materials.

Remember that antifungal drugs' side effects can cause many symptoms that are similar to Valley Fever. Some patients may need to take the drugs and endure the side effects for a lifetime. This can mean the drugs' side effects may continue long after Valley Fever has been put into remission.

Am I free and clear from the disease if I completely got over my Valley Fever infection (or if I was infected but never sickened by it)?

Valley Fever can activate or reactivate later in any patient's life whether the infection originally caused symptoms or not. This does not mean infected people should panic, simply that they should consider the possibility and alert their doctors if they have any of the symptoms later. See our Symptoms Chapter for more information.

Why has the incidence of Valley Fever been on the rise and how bad is the epidemic?

An excerpt from the 2/13/03 minutes of the Arizona State Senate Committee on Health follows:

> *"Dr. John Galgiani, Professor of Medicine, UA, and Director, Valley Fever Center for Excellence, distributed a handout (Attachment F) and provided an overview of the status of Valley Fever in Arizona. Currently, the State is experiencing an epidemic. [Years later, the epidemic is now far worse.] Although Valley Fever is a national problem, 65% of the cases are in Arizona. He stressed that Valley Fever could be used as an agent of bioterrorism. If the perceived risk of Valley Fever is not managed by education and research, businesses and tourists may go elsewhere.*
>
> *"Dr. Galgiani referred to this week's Center for Disease Control (CDC) Report, noting that Valley Fever is the fourth most commonly reported infectious disease to the Arizona Department of Health Services (DHS). The increase in reported infection is unexplained, but could possibly be linked to construction, climatic effects, and bioterroist [sic] attack.*
>
> *"...There is no clear explanation for the cause of the epidemic, which is in excess of the population growth...one in four college students are sick for up to four months. He pointed out the problems with current therapy, noting that less than 70% of patients respond to therapy. However, when therapy is stopped, relapses occur. He explained that indefinite therapy is expensive with lifetime therapy costing two-thirds of a million dollars for each patient."* [181]

The complete minutes are available here:
http://www.azleg.state.az.us/FormatDocument.asp?inDoc=/legt ext/46leg/1R/comm_min/Senate/0213+HEA%2EDOC.htm

The Valley Fever problem has become considerably worse. 2006's reported annual infections were so high they represented the worst Valley Fever epidemic in Arizona's recorded history, and 2007 was nearly as bad. This is not surprising. Nearly every previous year had also been the worst Valley Fever epidemic of its time for the past ten years.

Aside from Hepatitis C and sexually transmitted diseases, more people in Arizona were reported to have Valley Fever in 2007 than any other disease. This follows the trend from previous years.

Family: The Other Victims of Valley Fever

As valleyfeversurvivor.com's longtime readers already know, Valley Fever does not just affect the people who have contracted the disease. It can greatly alter the lives of their spouses, children, parents, grandparents, friends, co-workers, and even their pets.

A person who contracts Valley Fever may be in pain, have severe headaches and have chronic fatigue to name a few issues that must be dealt with. These issues may not go away for weeks, months, years, or they may never go away.

Valley Fever and Family Breakdowns

Imagine yourself as a man whose wife was "down for the count" due to ongoing Valley Fever symptoms. As the husband you might have to be responsible for cooking, cleaning, caring for your ill wife and working at your job. Care for your wife might be needed 24/7 and you may need to have a relative stay with her or hire a caretaker to be there at least five days a week. In some real world cases this scenario has gone on for years.

If you have young children, they will need to be cared for daily. They will no longer have their healthy mother to take care of them. The usual daily tasks of diaper changing, feeding children, getting them dressed, and playing with them would be out of the question for her. If the children are old enough to take care of themselves they may be required to help out at home and help care for their ill mother. That means they have less time for their friends and less personal freedom.

The children may be always worried about their mom or, as time goes by, some children resent having an ill mother. She may no longer be able to drive them places or attend their sporting events. Resentment over the focus on her needs may start to build and the relationship between the children and their mother could deteriorate. Sometimes if the children are old enough, they leave home so as not to be burdened by caring for their ill parent.

The husband of the ill wife may not fare much better. We know of too many families which started out with loving caregiving, but over time the healthy spouses lost their concerned and caring ways. In this example, a healthy husband can become annoyed and unhappy by what now seems to be a permanent health issue with his wife that he didn't bargain for. After all what about his sex life? They are not able to go dancing, backpacking, partying, or having "fun" anymore. The loving husband drifts further and further away and the marriage eventually breaks up leaving the Valley Fever sufferer alone, without support, and without any way to bring in an income, pay her bills or to get medical insurance.

This is not to suggest husbands infected with Valley Fever have it any easier. Switch "husband" with "wife" in the story above and it still paints a similar picture. Too many men have suffered a similar fate with wives who have grown impatient and calloused.

An example follows:

Dan F.
Contracted VF at 33 years old
San Diego, California

His initial questionnaire was concluded with this message:

THE LIFE I HAD WHICH WAS A GOOD ONE IS GONE... I'VE LOST EVERYTHING, TOO HARD TO PUT INTO WORDS ON A PAPER... FEEL FREE TO CALL ANYTIME... ONE ISSUE I HAVE IS SEVERE HAND SORENESS FROM MULTIPLE SURGERIES... TYPING IS DIFFICULT.

When we called him later, we were able to have a more complete story.

My Valley Fever started about five years ago and only recently have lesions started to occur. Six years ago I used to race motorcycles out in the desert in Imperial Valley. I am from Pennsylvania and about two summers ago I started racing out there and having a ball and one day my hands turned into the Pillsbury Dough Boy and they didn't know why. The doctors did a biopsy and found out it was Valley Fever.
I was a gas turbine mechanic, a jet engine kind of person. My employers thought I was trying to pull something over on them. They weren't willing to do any retraining or anything since I could not use my hands as before. Since I couldn't do my job (hold and work with heavy

wrenches and pull apart jet engines) they fired me. I couldn't get any support anywhere at all. When they hear Valley Fever they thought I should take some Tylenol and it would go away. That was what my boss' initial reaction was. My employer never believed I was sick.

Even though I had all the scars on my hands they just never believed me and fired me. I haven't been able to get a job and I don't have any insurance anymore. I have bouts where I can break out in lesions sometimes and my hands have been basically crippled due to all the surgeries I've had. If you look at me it doesn't look like there is anything wrong with me.

I was able to get diflucan through the Pfizer compassion program and I am still taking it. I take 800 mg a day and still get lesions. I've had three surgeries on one hand and two on the other. They pulled a whole small butter container's worth of cocci from my hands. The doctor said it was "rotten egg like." UC Davis identified the VF. I was also given lots of steroid shots, probably 20 of them. No one said not to have them with VF. To date I have had no sign of Valley Fever in my lungs—the nodules or scaring. It just disseminated elsewhere.

Valley Fever with all the stress and loss of job led to a divorce. I have two teenagers living here in California near me.

I've lost my family, I've lost my home, I've lost my job, my kids and everything. I live in a one bedroom apartment with no money. My parents send me money basically to stay alive. I have nothing left of my life since VF. I don't have any money and I am basically broke. I can't afford to see a doctor.

On behalf of everyone like me I appreciate what you are doing.

When we contacted him last, Dan was forced to give up his phone, computer, and anything that was considered a life. He simply could not afford to pay his bills. He was going to go back to the Midwest to live with his father.

Fortunately, not all cases are like this, but frustration can remain a constant part of Valley Fever.

Jenna C.
Stoneham, MA
Contracted VF at age 21 in Tucson, AZ

Valley Fever has drastically affected my family and myself. I was the first person diagnosed in my family. Before Valley Fever I was extremely healthy with the occasional sinus infection due to allergies. I now have joint pain, headaches, dizziness, problems breathing, high fevers and an inability to focus and remember things.

I had symptoms of Valley Fever starting in 1997 but wasn't diagnosed until a year later. After several visits to the doctors and by the third visit to the ER, a student doctor noticed the red bumps all over my legs accompanied by massive swelling in my feet, ankles and legs. He immediately did blood work and told me that I had Valley Fever. I didn't know about titer levels then. I was given an anti-inflammatory to reduce the swelling and pain killers for my legs. My doctors were of no help and I was told that the VF would go away on its own. A year later, I was able to reduce the symptoms completely by moving to the New England area and sleeping weekends at a time.

I still have outbreaks including the one that has brought me to the internet searching for more information so I can educate my doctors. It is frustrating that there is such a gap in the medical community regarding this disease and a lack of understanding or compassion when you are diagnosed with Valley Fever.

I've met people who have said they have had reoccurring outbreaks of VF and that it has drastically changed their lives. I know it has changed my life at 21. Once a health enthusiast I was too tired to even walk around my neighborhood. Some days I was too tired to even get out of bed.

In my last semester of school before I graduate, I have recently felt the symptoms return and fear the doctor's visits I know I am going to have to endure.

Since I was first diagnosed, my family dog was diagnosed. Soon after that my Dad became extremely ill with VF too. I was able to direct him to sites so that he could educate his doctors. He still lives with VF in the Tucson area and has had to take several months off of work last year. In fact, his short term disability insurance with MetLife refused to pay his claim because they did not believe VF was a serious disease.

I am very passionate about the subject of Valley Fever not only because it has impacted my life in such a personal way, but because so many people do not understand the implications that come with living with such a disease.

Children with Valley Fever

If it isn't bad enough when a parent contracts Valley Fever, it is even worse when a child is sickened with this disease. Most parents will tell you that the loss of a child is far more devastating emotionally than the loss of a parent or a spouse. A 2006 study using the 2002 National Inpatient Sample showed an 8.5% death rate nationally for children hospitalized with Valley Fever.[49] In our opinion this is totally unacceptable.

Children who live with severe and chronic Valley Fever conditions face many hardships and might require constant care. If a child contracts this disease it may mean a loss of income from the caregiver whose schedule could revolve around doctor appointments and health care. It could create financial hardships and strain relationships between the caregiver and the other spouse or children in the family. Everything can change drastically.   If the caregiver is a single parent, it can be a financial catastrophe.

Depending on the severity of the infection, a child with Valley Fever may no longer be able to take care of him or herself for quite some time.   Valley Fever's symptoms can also keep a child from playing with friends or socializing.   Friends leave, not understanding what is happening and even worry about if they can "catch" Valley Fever like a cold.

The child becomes more isolated.   After a while, even siblings may get tired of their brother or sister always being sick, going to doctors or to the hospital, and their mother, father, or both being unable to be there for the healthy children in the family.

Valley Fever can strain the family unit to the breaking point, and has sometimes split up families.

Conflict Outside the Family

All too often, friends and co-workers also fade away with their support.   They frequently believe the person with Valley Fever should be "better by now," mainly because they do not have the slightest understanding of this incurable disease.   They cannot seem to grasp that this is the most virulent fungal parasite known to man and is destroying the person from the inside out.

A co-worker or friend may have experienced an initially mild case of Valley Fever that had gone into remission.   He or she might not understand why anyone else with the same disease could be suffering so terribly.   People like this might even believe the severe Valley Fever case is psychosomatic instead, as some uninformed doctors have (continue reading below and also read our Testing and Diagnosis Chapter for more information).

People with Valley Fever may look fine on the outside but are being ravaged on the inside.   In some cases, friends and family are misinformed and afraid that the person may be contagious so they stay away.   In other cases it is merely a lack of knowledge, lack of understanding, lack of compassion, or complete selfishness.

Many people lose their jobs as a result of being too tired and unable to complete their assignments.   Some Valley Fever patients find that their memory is not as good as it was,[234] making

them unable to do the complicated or technical job they once
had. This often happens to men but of course can happen to
women as well. In survivors' telephone and e-mail contact with
us, they commonly referred to it as "brain fog."

When the breadwinner loses his or her job, the family's
health insurance can be lost when it is most desperately needed.
The medications that treat Valley Fever are expensive, and doctor
visits and hospital stays are very costly. Most families are
devastated if they are caught without health insurance at this
time.

Military men and women also pay a big price for being in
endemic zones and contracting Valley Fever. We know of men
that contracted this disease while serving their country while they
were in their twenties and have never been able to be an active
father to their children as a result of this disease. The children
lose out as well as the father and mother.

Many of our readers with chronic or disseminated Valley
Fever have told similar stories. Simple activities like walking up
stairs or walking across the street to the mailbox take on new
meaning when extreme fatigue has set in. A commonly repeated
question is "when will this fatigue go away?"

For many, everyday tasks like vacuuming have become far
too much effort to contemplate. Employment suffers when
those with Valley Fever go to work, do poorly at their job, and go
home immediately to sleep 14 hours or more. Others are unable
to work or sleep due to chronic pain or breathing difficulties.

Valley Fever may cause lesions that can only be
removed by amputations and surgeries.[69, 88, 211] When lesions
from Valley Fever are plainly visible, "the result may be
shocking deformity and disfigurement."[75]

There are physical difficulties and disfigurements to
contend with as well. There is a young woman in the military
in California who contacted us and mentioned that she needed
to have a thumb removed after several surgeries were
unsuccessful in stopping the spread of Valley Fever in her
hand.

Depression

The realization of these changes can bring an extreme depth of despair as people recognize their old way of living is gone forever. This can be compounded by unsympathetic friends, family, and employers who are sometimes angry at the person with Valley Fever and declare he or she should just "get over it," as if anyone with this disease would not want their suffering to go away.

Depression often sets in when people realize they will never be the same active person they were prior to their Valley Fever. In addition, some Valley Fever sufferers think about suicide. Several people have contacted us seriously contemplating ending their lives due to this disease. We have heard from someone who believed her sister with Valley Fever committed suicide due to the pain and suffering from the disease and a lack of hope from doctors who wouldn't take Valley Fever seriously. The seriousness of this possibility should not be overlooked.

There is one important thing that we need to say regarding the thoughts of suicide or just wishing to die so the suffering will end:

Please, never give up! As long as there is life there is always hope and coming from experience I know that there are miracles performed every day. If you need someone to talk with about your severe depression make sure you do so. Every life is worth saving. You can always write to me and I will be there for you to help you through your very difficult time.

Some doctors don't help in this matter by telling the infected person that "you should be feeling better by now" or that all the fatigue, aches, pains, and other symptoms are "all in your head" and recommending a psychiatrist rather than further medical care. These comments, unfortunately, show a lack of knowledge by the physician for the nuances of this disease. When statements like these are heard by a family member who also doesn't know any better, it creates even less understanding and support for the person with Valley Fever.

Fortunately, not all families, friends, co-workers, and physicians react this way. There are many loving and caring families that stand by their beloved family member who is infected with the fungal parasite that causes Valley Fever. The strength, love and support of people around those afflicted by coccidioidomycosis are of utmost importance. The depression that many Valley Fever sufferers experience from this disease is difficult enough and quite understandable.

How People Can Be Affected

Sonny W.
Contracted VF at 43 years old
Salinas, California

Life is at a slower pace. I get tired very easily now. I am on 800mg of Fluconazole a day for life. I was out two and a half years from work...but the main boss worked with me. I just stumbled through the tired feeling and retired ASAP. Like the head nurse told me at the hospital before they released me "Listen to your body." I pace myself and try not to get sick again. I do hope there will be a cure in the future.

Rebecca R. (written by her mother)
Contracted VF as a one year old
Simi Valley, California

I lost work and pay with my husband who needed to care for our other two children and help me. We are anxious and afraid it will come back. Children's Hospital is a wonderful place to get well, however, they are not very good at people skills or communication between departments which made Rebecca's stay unnecessarily much longer. We were never kept aware of what was going on with her and were treated like ones who were just in the way. Rebecca had no previous illnesses.

Henry C.
Contracted VF at 19 years old
Bakersfield, California

With my sickness and being so young it's really hard. I can't work so I feel I've become a burden on my family and friends with needs for money due to medicine and doctor visits.

Debbie
Contracted VF at 44 years old
Porterville, California

Lost my job of 26 years due to ongoing symptoms of VF and am considered disabled now. I have been diagnosed with Fibromyalgia/Chronic Fatigue Syndrome, high cholesterol and depression. I have wheezing, headaches, vision problems, malaise, nausea, muscle aches, muscle stiffness, joint pain, joint swelling, joint stiffness, leg swelling, foot swelling, ankle swelling, short term memory loss, mental fatigue, loss of stamina and continue to tire quickly and easily.

My entire way of life changed seemingly overnight. I was very physically active, healthy, fiercely independent and quite capable of caring for myself my entire life. I was in the process of fixing up my house to sell and "move up" since I had recently received a promotion. Everything stopped...plans, dreams, goals, my music and other hobbies. I was medically retired out of my job because I was no longer strong enough or healthy enough to continue.

I now have to have help with just about everything; laundry, cooking, driving, grocery shopping, paying bills, cleaning house and what friends or family won't help me with, I have to pay for, such as lawn and yard care, which I always preferred to do myself before being stricken down with Valley Fever.

I'm mostly housebound now. It is difficult to keep social contacts and appointments. I am in excruciating, ever-present relentless pain and burning in just about every muscle and joint in my body. This pain has been here for almost 4 years. The intensity of the pain waxes and wanes, but there's never a day or night that it's not with me. Loss of independence and vitality is the greatest loss of all due to Valley Fever and it doesn't look as though I'm going to get back 100% any time soon.

Rachel B.
Contracted VF at 27 years old
Gilbert, AZ

It was a nightmare. My husband worked 11+ hours a day and I had no family around. He lost some work on my BAD days. Trying to take care of my 4 kids was impossible. I would have NEVER made it if it weren't for members of my church stepping in and taking care of my kids and house and family while I tried to rest the best I could. I thought my life was never going to be normal again. I feel so blessed that I am back to normal and hope nothing surfaces again.

I fear for my kids though. I do NOT want my kids to EVER go through what I went through. I have even thought about dropping EVERYTHING we have here to move away from all areas it is possible to get VF.

Shelley W.
Contracted VF at 41 years old
Phoenix, Arizona

I have had Valley Fever for over a year. I have been shuffled from doctor to doctor with no concrete treatment plan in place as of yet. My family doctor is finally sending me to an Infectious Disease doc next week. Three months ago this same ID doc treated me over the phone with a prescription of Sporanox. He stated that I had a "hole" in my immune system where I am not able to fight the disease. He told me to take the medicine the rest of my life. I have had three short remissions in the past year but the disease keeps coming back.

I have continuing lung pain with no improvement on the same spot in my lung for over a year. I still have numerous non-calcified nodules in my right upper lung.

My family has been supportive and helpful. I am lucky that my children are teenagers and are able to fend for themselves at home. There are many days where I come home from work and go straight to bed.

Prior to becoming an accountant seven years ago, I worked in the emergency room at a Phoenix hospital. I was aware of VF but never imagined it to be such a severe disease. The more people I talk to I hear of very bad cases.

Launa P.
Contracted VF at 37 years old
Glendale, Arizona

I was very healthy (I only had an occasional cold or flu) prior to contracting VF. I lost my job, could not keep up with the hours. By losing my job I lost my insurance. I finally got another job with insurance. The insurance company put me on "probation" for 3 months, charged more due to the "pre-existing condition." I was laid off from that job. I lost my house that I owned as I needed meds and my life was more important to me than owning a house. The medication is more than I can afford at this time in my life as I am a single woman raising two children. From time to time my doctor has been able to give me samples of the Diflucan, which has been wonderful. I can not afford the medication and I am out and feeling the effects again. The achiness in my body is eased some by Ibuprofen. I drink a lot of caffeine to get through the work day and the time my children need from me daily.

This disease has helped me see life a little differently. I appreciate things much more and have learned to focus on more important things, such as spending time with my kids and not worrying about how the house is going to get cleaned when I am too tired. My children have learned to appreciate health, theirs and others. It has helped them learn compassion. There are up sides to all negatives, perhaps mine was to learn how to slow down and enjoy life more. However, I don't know what more I can give up as the financial burden has become too much.

Stress seems to make the illness worse and it is not easy to not stress when without the medication I get so ill...there is not enough money to pay for the medication. It's a crazy circle. I don't know where to turn, what to do. I want to live a life without pain, exhaustion and without financial strain. I want to be able to get health insurance without complication.

James J.
Contracted VF at 42 years old
Atlanta, Georgia

I suffer from depression. I have calcifications, scarring on my face, arms and back. I have no energy. Valley Fever has devastated me emotionally, spiritually, physically and financially.

Karen Bert, on behalf of her son Tyson Paul
Kern County, CA
Sun, April 13, 2003

My 19 year old son Tyson, was diagnosed with Valley Fever in January 2003. His VF had also disseminated into his bones which had eaten away at his hip bones and part of his lumbar spine. He was told to avoid falls because his bones were so brittle. Our worse fears happened when he fell going to the bathroom. He broke his lumbar 5, landing him in the hospital for fifteen days.

Tyson has had a rough time but we can finally see a light at the end of the tunnel. He is currently on Ampho IV three times a week. I can't begin to tell you how Valley Fever has affected my family. We have had a very rough four months. The doctor says he has probably had this for at least six months prior.

I can only thank God for watching over him. Tyson's titer was a 1:512 when we started out. At the last test it was a 1:248. He was born in Kern County and is an African American male with asthma and sickle cell trait, but was never really sick before contracting VF.

October 2007 Update

Tyson Paul is in his fourth year of college. He is on daily medication but holding his own. We were very pleased to hear from his mother Karen that he is doing so much better.

This is truly a story of faith and hope. We all thank God for Tyson's recovery and we wish him much success, health and happiness in the future.

An Important Message for Family and Friends of Every Valley Fever Survivor

It is difficult to watch someone you love and care about be ill and in pain. As time goes by, many Valley Fever Survivors start to feel somewhat better but far from the way they used to be health-wise.

As a spouse, child, co-worker or friend of that person, you are likely to ask the following questions. For simplicity, only female pronouns were used below, but these questions have been routinely asked of male and female Valley Fever victims:

- Why doesn't she stop complaining and crying?
- Why doesn't she get back to work and stop being lazy?
- Why doesn't she stop sleeping so much?
- Why doesn't she stop being depressed and just snap out of it?
- Why isn't she as outgoing and fun to be with anymore?
- Why hasn't she gone on with her life and get back to all the things she did before her Valley Fever?

Unfortunately, the answer to all those questions is that Valley Fever can change lives permanently. Survivors would be very happy to go back to doing everything they did before their Valley Fever but are just not capable of it.

While some family members start with empathy for the person with Valley Fever, we often hear that they lose this empathy as the sickness wears on. Many either do not understand or do not want to believe that Valley Fever can become chronic and possibly permanently debilitating. Fatigue can become a daily fact of life for many with Valley Fever.

Since Valley Fever can become dormant and reactivate at any time, the one living with this incurable disease is obviously unhappy about it. Wouldn't you be?

If it does become dormant that does not mean that the person will have their previous energy level return or be capable of all the tasks they could handle prior to Valley Fever. Their lives may be changed forever.

Unsuspecting tourists, university students, retirees and businesses are lured to the Southwest without any knowledge, much less a warning that this severe disease even exists. Who would ever imagine the most virulent fungus known to man could live and thrive in the desert? Too many residents are misinformed as well because they have been mistakenly led to believe Valley Fever was a benign disease and that it could only happen to people who were sick with other diseases or people who work in the dust like construction workers or farmers. Anyone at any health level, at any age, can contract a serious, chronic or deadly case of Valley Fever.

This ongoing epidemic has been kept a "local secret" for decades.[100] It is estimated that over 400,000 people have contracted VF in 2006 and that nearly as many people were infected in 2007. Many of them have no idea that it is in their body as they have been misdiagnosed or it has not activated yet. It is horrifying and frustrating that from all these infections, only 2% or less are diagnosed accurately.[19, 244]

Valley Fever can kill, but it can also affect its survivors for a lifetime. It can disseminate to the eyes where it can cause blindness and possibly require the removal of an infected eye. Valley Fever can attack any organ or limb in the body to cause lesions, chronic pain, and to require amputations. Some cases can necessitate surgical removal of an infected lung, or the disease can mimic the appearance of lung cancer and lead to surgical removals that otherwise may not have been necessary. Valley Fever can cause facial lesions that leave permanent scaring and disfigurement. In the most lethal variety of the disease it can attack the lining of the brain (meninges), possibly making its victims lose their mental faculties or have permanent brain damage. Valley Fever can infect the bones and joints, causing chronic debilitation, pain, and resulting in the need for joint fusions or amputations.

The following two pages have photographs that show some of the worst outward disfigurement that Valley Fever can cause. While its effects on the outside are horrific, it is worth remembering that many Valley Fever patients are suffering with lesions like these on the inside.

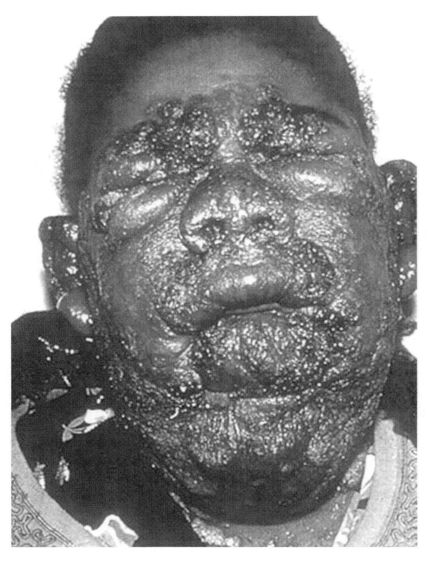

This Valley Fever victim has cutaneous lesions on most of his face and neck. One can only imagine the suffering and pain this man experienced. When people are fortunate enough not to have outwardly visible lesions, doctors, family, and friends often do not realize the horrors that may be happening on the inside of the body. Image courtesy of Dr. John W. Rippon.

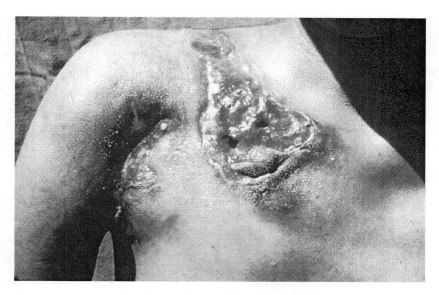

The picture above shows an ulcerated plaque caused by Valley Fever. Image courtesy of Dr. John W. Rippon.

Too many people with Valley Fever have become wheelchair bound as a result of disseminated spinal lesions or from having too many spinal taps. Too many people need shunts to be surgically implanted into their skulls to receive amphotericin B injections to kill cocci in their cerebrospinal fluid. The antifungal drugs can have terrible side effects, but may need to be taken for a lifetime since patients who stopped taking the drugs relapsed within a year in 75% of cases.[48] These antifungal drugs are not cures since they only bring the population of cocci down. The hope is that the patient's immune system can take over and cause these rapidly multiplying fungal parasites to go dormant in the body.

Valley Fever can cause dangerous inflammation and lesions in virtually any part of the human body. In men it can infect the prostate and testicles, causing removal of the infected organs. If a young woman of childbearing age has to remain on lifelong antifungal drugs to keep the disease at bay, she may be told she can never have children.

I have heard from too many people and their families that lost their homes, jobs, health insurance, and their ability to enjoy life because of inhaling a *Coccidioides* sp. spore. Only you can decide what risks you are willing to take with your health and your family's health, but you need to know all the facts about the disease and the endemic areas in order to make an informed decision. Tragically, most people only learn about Valley Fever after they are infected with it.

We hope those of you reading this book understand a little more about the horrendous disease your loved one has contracted, and will be there for them to help them through the most difficult health issue they may ever face.

It is important for all those around a person suffering with Valley Fever to have more empathy. The changes in that person's behavior may be life altering for you, but imagine how much worse it is for the person with this disease. Please remember that this is the only fungal parasite regulated by two antiterrorism laws and is the most virulent fungus known to man. It should be expected to make a big impact on an infected person's life.

Your support and compassion can mean everything to those suffering with Valley Fever. Please keep your mind and heart open to understanding what your loved one with Valley Fever has to endure.

If you are living in an endemic zone or visit an endemic zone it is also possible that you can inhale an air dispersed spore and contract this disease yourself. It doesn't matter how healthy you were prior to Valley Fever but how healthy you are after contracting Valley Fever—and if you are already infected, whether and how Valley Fever reactivates.

The only way to stop this epidemic is with a vaccine and cure. Please read Appendix A: Organizations and Internet Resources to find out how you can help to make this happen.

Thank you for caring. We wish all Valley Fever Survivors and their family and friends love, understanding, and peace through their trying experiences with this disease.

What You Need to Know Before You See a Doctor

It always pays to have as much information as possible about the journey to a successful diagnosis, whether coccidioidomycosis or any other disease is involved.

This chapter describes the possible consequences of many ordinary Valley Fever tests and the steps patients can take to ensure the finest medical care. Medical tragedies have proven this information to be necessary.

At A Glance

- Certain tests like lumbar punctures (spinal taps), MRIs using certain contrast agents, and CT scans can pose serious health risks.
- From patients' experiences, doctors do not always inform their patients when they intend to conduct frequent and dangerous tests on the progress of their treatment. Patients may need to ask about this ahead of time and may not want to have such frequent testing.
- When visiting a doctor, patients should be prepared with a list of questions.
- Patients should always double check that the medication they receive is exactly what it should be.
- The doctors that most commonly treat Valley Fever patients specialize in pulmonary (lung) conditions or infectious diseases.
- You are your own best advocate and if you are not satisfied with your current physicians, do not hesitate to find new ones.

Risks Associated with Some Tests and Treatments

It is a cliché that a cure can be worse than a disease. Even though there presently is no cure for Valley Fever, some tests can be worse than the disease, or at least just as bad. Lumbar punctures (commonly known as spinal taps) and some imaging tests can cause agony patients had never even imagined.

The Danger of Spinal Taps

When spinal taps are taken, amphotericin B infusions are given, or other spinal punctures occur, the spine's sensitive tissue can be irritated. This irritation can cause nerves to stick together or be damaged. The end result can be spinal scarring that causes severe, chronic, lifelong pain. This is a condition known as arachnoiditis.

The inflammation from spinal irritants "can sometimes lead to the formation of scar tissue and adhesions, which cause the spinal nerves to 'stick' together. If arachnoiditis begins to interfere with the function of one or more of these nerves, it can cause a number of symptoms, including numbness, tingling, and a characteristic stinging and burning pain in the lower back or legs. Some people with arachnoiditis will have debilitating muscle cramps, twitches, or spasms. It may also affect bladder, bowel, and sexual function. In severe cases, arachnoiditis may cause paralysis of the lower limbs."[188]

Except for the most severe cases, there is no reason to have, for example, weekly spinal taps to check a *Coccidioides* titer in the cerebrospinal fluid. While this might be done in a critical case, some patients reported excessively frequent testing was done as a result of their doctors' research programs.

Plotting frequent "data points" may be interesting when researchers write their reports, but most patients whose spines are repeatedly punctured are unlikely to care about medical journals; they'll only care about how much they hurt. Further, the extra ink their doctors are able to print will be of little comfort if the spinal taps cause arachnoiditis and leave the patient with a lifetime of chronic spinal pain or paralysis.

Spinal taps for testing are often taken six weeks apart or longer. However, more frequent testing might be necessary for some patients. With this in mind, ask that your spine only be punctured for the testing and medication you absolutely need. Ask your doctor whether it would be acceptable for spinal taps to be taken less often. This advice came to us from a medical professional in the endemic areas and by patients who tragically suffered paralysis as a result of their spinal taps.

Learn from Experience with Spinal Taps

Not every spinal problem results in irreversible paralysis or ongoing pain, so it is important for patients to know when they can take action to improve their lives. At our www.valleyfeversurvivor.com message board, a poster with the screen name Patti1010 shared the following information. Everyone needs to be vigilant with their medical care, and her story demonstrates this need more clearly than any simple warning could.

In her story Patti uses the technical term "lumbar puncture" and abbreviates it as LP rather than using "spinal tap."

I don't want to create any more anxiety than already exists when dealing with this disease but I had an experience with a lumbar puncture that I wanted to share so hopefully you don't share the same problems. Before proceeding I want to make sure it's understood that not all LPs have the same complications. My experience may not be the same as the next 100 people to have an LP but I thought it would be informative and I wish I had known ahead of time.

I had put off the LP because I thought it would hurt. In truth, it was really not that big a deal. The poke is about 10 seconds of—can't so much say pain as the sting of a needle. The only other issue I felt was the funky nerve pain that shot down the leg. Again, it wasn't awful, and the doctor would move the needle so it was momentary. That happened on a Friday morning.

It's of utmost importance not to move and lay as flat as possible after the procedure for several hours. I was kept at the hospital for about 2-3 hours and there I did fine. I went home and kept up with the directions of laying flat but trying to take in caffeinated fluids that would help. 24 hours later, I thought I was doing much better. The headache had been bearable and it had actually gone away.

Sunday morning I woke with this massive head pain. I called my doctor who explained that I should go to the ER and mention that I might need a blood patch. For those of you who don't know—a blood patch is a fix in which they take some of your own blood and inject it into the LP site to close the hole leaking the spinal fluid which is why you have the massive head pain.

The ER doctor came in and told me he didn't really understand why my doctor would have said I needed a blood patch. That requires an anesthesiologist and is a "procedure" by itself. That's not usually done for 7 days post LP. He claimed that some IV caffeine is usually warranted and of course meds for the pain. My experience only got worse. I was vomiting and still had pain. I was sent home with the declaration that I was given everything that could be done. My pain had lessened and was bearable but I was practically unconscious and retching regularly.

The next day the pain was worse. I went to another ER on my primary doctor's suggestion that they would do something to help. All they did was give me drugs that completely knocked me out. I apparently was poured into my car and sent home to sleep it off. I slept 21 straight hours. I guess if I was in pain I wouldn't have known it. I woke up on Thursday, which was incidentally Thanksgiving Day still in pain. My husband called the primary care doctor and pleaded with him to tell him what to do. He called back shortly thereafter, bless him, and explained what to tell the ER.

This is where my advice comes in...he said to tell them you want an anesthesiologist consult for the blood patch. If not they'll just give you drugs to mitigate the pain as best they can. I did some research on the blood patch procedure and yes, although it is a "procedure" and requires an anesthesiologist, the pain can be alleviated completely in 20 minutes. It is less common for doctors to automatically order the consult and you may have to insist on it.

It has to be an individual decision of course. In my case the pain on a scale of 10 was 9 to 12. In hindsight, I lost 4 unnecessary days due to the pain. I was incoherent a majority of the time, and that in itself is a real issue for me. The additional disappointment of having to cancel making Thanksgiving dinner only made it worse. The reality that I could have been pain-free all that time made me so angry.

It's not a given that all lumbar punctures cause the headache and not always does it have the same intensity so I don't want to scare anyone away from the procedure if you need it. I would do it again if I had to with someone standing by to make sure I had the blood patch if it happened again. I wanted to make sure you are informed of your right to have the pain alleviated in short order and not have doctors making the decisions for you. As with every procedure there are risks, but I took a risk as well having the doctors pump more and more pain meds in, causing a temporary arrhythmia.

Dangerous Radiation from CT Scans

Doctors often call for CT scans to help diagnose their patients' illnesses. Perhaps this occurs too often, since this method of imaging internal organs use potentially dangerous levels of radiation. Even low doses of radiation measured in millisieverts (mSv) may cause cancer.

"Many studies have shown that organ doses associated with routine diagnostic CT scans are similar to the low-dose range of radiation received by atomic-bomb survivors. The FDA estimates that a CT examination with an effective dose of 10 mSv may be associated with an increased chance of developing fatal cancer for approximately one patient in 2000, whereas the BEIR [Biologic Effects of Ionizing Radiation] VII lifetime risk model predicts that with the same low-dose radiation, approximately one individual in 1000 will develop cancer."[222]

PET scans and CT scans can provide from 100 to 1000 times as much radiation as a single simple x-ray. CT scans account for 67% of medical radiation overall, and the cancer risks of radioactive exposure at one time extend throughout a patient's life. Even so, soft tissue like the lungs and heart may have their problems diagnosed easier with a CT scan than with some other, less radioactive, methods.[222]

The dose of radiation should also be proportioned to the size of the patient because the effect of any given dose is stronger on a smaller person than a larger one. Aside from their smaller size, children face additional risks from CT scans. "Because they have more rapidly dividing cells than adults and have longer life expectancy, the odds that children will develop cancers from x-ray radiation may be significantly higher than adults."[4]

The FDA released a public health notification about the specific dangers of medical radiation exposure to children and small adults in 2001. This notification mentioned that many medical personnel are not aware of patient overexposures. With a conventional x-ray the look of an overexposed image is obvious, but an image from a CT scan may look fine even when the patient has been overexposed. "Several recent articles stress that it is important to use the lowest radiation dose necessary to provide an image from which an accurate diagnosis can be made, and that significant dose reductions can be achieved without compromising clinical efficacy."[82] Like many warnings, it may take time before this becomes fully institutionalized.

It has been repeatedly suggested that radiation exposures be kept "as low as reasonably achievable" as a general guideline for all patients.[82,222] In addition, the FDA made specific recommendations to optimize settings of CT equipment and reduce exposures. One of these recommendations follows:

"Eliminate inappropriate referrals for CT. In some cases, conventional radiography, sonography, or magnetic resonance imaging (MRI) can be just as effective as CT, and with lower radiation exposure. Most conventional x-ray units deliver less ionizing radiation than CT systems, and sonography and MRI systems deliver no x-ray radiation at all. It is important to triage these examinations to eliminate inappropriate referrals or to utilize procedures with less or no ionizing radiation."[82]

Some patients who had Valley Fever for a long time and were later diagnosed with cancer wonder whether VF could have caused their cancer. While coccidioidomycosis has frequently been misdiagnosed as cancer, it is not known to cause cancer on its own.   However, if enough CT scans were used to evaluate Valley Fever lesions, and sufficiently dangerous radioactive exposures occurred, the testing and monitoring of Valley Fever could have caused cancer.

The doctors who frequently use radiology may find the FDA's public health notification very useful, and patients may wish to read this so they can ask questions before receiving an unnecessary dose of radiation.

http://www.fda.gov/cdrh/safety/110201-ct.html

MRI Dangers

MRI procedures use magnetism instead of radiation. This means they may be safer than CT scans in some cases, but not every case. Some MRIs will not require that unusual substances are given to patients, while others may need an injection that will help improve the clarity of the pictures. A gadolinium-based contrast agent can make these pictures clearer, but it can also harm the patient.

In 2006, the FDA highlighted the danger of gadolinium-based contrast agents (GBCA). Patients with renal insufficiency (kidneys that are not filtering waste products properly) and patients at and near the time of their liver transplantation surgeries (with even slight renal insufficiency) are at risk. People from both groups who had taken GBCAs to enhance their MRIs had an enhanced risk of a condition called nephrogenic systemic fibrosis.

A fibrosis is the excess buildup of fibrous connective material (like scars) within the body. Nephrogenic systemic fibrosis can cause an excess buildup of fibrous tissue anywhere in the body, particularly the skin and connective tissues.

"The skin thickening may inhibit flexion and extension of joints resulting in contractures [inabilities to stretch muscles]. In addition, patients may develop widespread fibrosis of other organs. A skin biopsy is necessary to confirm the diagnosis. The condition may be debilitating or cause death. Its cause is unknown and there is no consistently successful treatment."[83]

The FDA report recognized this risk of using GBCAs in people with kidney insufficiencies so it recommended to doctors that for "these patients, avoid the use of a GBCA unless the diagnostic information is essential and not available with non-contrast enhanced magnetic resonance imaging. [Nephrogenic systemic fibrosis] may result in fatal or debilitating systemic fibrosis."[83] Another article mentioned that doctors might have to weigh the dangers of CT scans against the dangers of a GBCA used in an MRI in order to have the most effective and least harmful test for their patient.[146]

Since Valley Fever and the drugs that treat it can both harm the kidneys, this is a worthwhile consideration for doctors and patients alike. The FDA's information is available at this Internet link:

http://www.fda.gov/CDER/drug/InfoSheets/HCP/gcca_2007_05.htm

The MRI procedure is intended to help doctors diagnose the patient better; not to cripple the patient's ability to move their arms and legs, put them into a wheelchair, have their organs malfunction, and kill them.

If you must have an MRI, ask if you absolutely need to be given a gadolinium-based contrast agent. If your doctor says yes, ask whether there are any alternatives, especially if there is any question about the strength of your kidney function.

It is said that laws are written on dead men's chests, and the same could certainly be said of updates to any medical procedure. After all, nephrogenic systemic fibrosis "can develop quickly, leading to the need for a wheelchair within weeks of the first symptoms."[213]

As one might expect, with the potential for a simple test to turn into a debilitating or deadly nightmare, ample opportunities for legal action arise.

A simple Internet search for "nephrogenic systemic fibrosis" and "lawsuit" is an eye opening experience for anyone considering an MRI with a GBCA. A small sampling of these law firms' web sites follows, and many others can quickly be found in an Internet search. We are not associated with or advocating use of these law firms in any way. We are simply using the URLs as examples of the legal assistance that is available:

http://www.gadolinium-mri.com/
http://www.gadoliniumlawyers.com/
http://www.reyeslaw.com/dangerous-drugs/gadolinium.asp
http://www.youhavealawyer.com/gadolinium/gadolinium-side-effects.html

Helpful Hints for Your Doctor Visits

You must take charge of your medical care. If you or a loved one must go to a doctor, there are a few things you will need to consider right away:

Meet the Staff

If the doctor's staff is cold, uncommunicative, and slow to respond, this often reflects the way the doctor will respond. If you have to search for a new doctor, contact the staff and consider their attitude and behavior as a possible preview of the doctor's attitude and behavior.

Prepare your Questions

A few days before your visit, write a list of every question you might want to ask your doctor during your visit. Check your list each day to see if there are any other questions you might add, or if you are able to get the information sooner, perhaps by phone. When trying to think of questions, a part of your preparation should include reading this book from cover to cover. This way, if you are prescribed 2000mg/d of fluconazole, for example, the Drugs and Treatment Chapter would inform you that it is an unusually high dose and that you might want to ask specific questions about your treatment.

Do not expect that you can memorize all your questions or the doctor's specific responses, because it is easy to become emotional and distracted with health matters. Consequently, when you call to make the appointment, ask if there is any objection to bringing an audio recorder; if the staff or doctors are afraid to have your appointment recorded, you may wish to find an office that is more accommodating. Bring an audio recorder or a pad and pencil with you to ensure you can accurately record the doctor's comments.

During your appointment with the doctor, make sure every question on your list is answered to your satisfaction, write the answers down, and take the written answers home with you. Even if you have an audio recording of the conversation, writing the answers on paper may make them more accessible to you later.

It may also be helpful to bring someone with you who would record the meeting and take notes for you. Review your questions and concerns with your friend before your medical visit. The review helps because he or she may remember to ask a question if you missed something in your notes when listening to the doctor. Your friend may also help by coming up with new questions for you.

In your list of questions, be sure to ask about some of the specific items below.

Request Copies of All Your Records

After every visit with a medical practitioner, ask for copies of all the additional medical records that were generated from that visit. Some doctors may be hesitant to do so, believing they are being set up for a lawsuit, but explain to them that you want to keep track of everything that is happening with your health and that a copy of their medical documentation is critical to that end.

Hospitals and doctors' offices may charge copying fees. We have heard of 10 or 11 cents per page; it may be higher or lower in your doctor's office, and it may or may not be covered by insurance. You will also want copies of all imaging tests, including CT scans and x-rays as a part of your complete documentation. Further explanation appears later in this chapter.

Some documents such as lab reports will not be available by the time your visit is finished, so ask when to expect the documents to be ready. Keep a file and log book of every document that you have and a list of when other documents are expected. You may have to ask more than once for your documents, but **always remember you have a legal right to see everything that is written about your case.** Note in your log book the date and time that you request a document and when it is received.

Hopefully you and your doctor will have open communication about your health care. Should you get into a situation with an uncooperative doctor's office, a lawyer ultimately may be necessary to acquire your medical documents. Your log records will show that you had no other choice due to the lack of cooperation from the doctor or his staff.

If your medical practitioners are not cooperating, it may be because they are understaffed and the few workers there do not believe they have time to make copies, they may have difficulties with their staff (punctuality, competence, etc.), or they may be trying to hide a medical mistake to avoid a malpractice suit. In any of these cases, this is a bad sign and you may wish to seek another physician.

Protection Against the Cancer Misdiagnosis

Valley Fever's lung nodules have frequently been misdiagnosed as lung cancer. The Arizona Respiratory Center recommends patients keep copies of x-rays with Valley Fever nodules so the nodules are not misdiagnosed as lung cancer later. If your chest x-rays (or other imaging tests like CT or PET scans) seem to show lung cancer and you have at some time lived in, visited, or received packages from an endemic region, you may wish to have yourself checked for Valley Fever. When surgery is suggested under these circumstances, you may wish to get a second opinion as to whether the lung cancer diagnosis is accurate before surgery.

Just because a doctor sees a lung nodule on a chest x-ray, it does not necessarily mean the patient has Valley Fever. However, the misdiagnosis of cancer is routinely given to Valley Fever patients. Sometimes they only discover that the lesion was from *Coccidioides* instead of cancer after the lesion and a large part of a lung was surgically removed and biopsied. If a doctor suspects cancer when Valley Fever is a possibility, previously taken x-rays and other imaging scans can help patients to avoid a lot of pain and suffering as well as the unnecessary surgeries to remove internal organs.

The fact that the disease has so many faces has made it difficult to diagnose, but one of the best ways has been with a travel history. If patients had been through or near California's San Joaquin Valley, Arizona, northwestern Mexico and other endemic areas, that information can be a Valley Fever tip-off to alert suspicious doctors—especially if the symptoms began in the typical 1–4 week incubation period. If your doctor has not inquired into your travel history, mention it and ask about the possibility of endemic diseases. This may help to diagnose coccidioidomycosis or perhaps another travel-related disease.

Ask About Sanitation Procedures

"Health care personnel are always on the go which sometimes makes handwashing with soap and water difficult,"[235] and this contributes to the nearly 2 million patients who are infected in hospitals each year. Nearly 100,000 are estimated to die annually as a result of these accidental in-hospital infections.[40] CDC Director Julie Gerberding said "Clean hands are the single most important factor in preventing the spread of dangerous germs and antibiotic resistance in health care settings."[104]

There are always plenty of sinks and antiseptic hand sanitizers in a hospital, so no doctor should ever examine you without clean hands or medical instruments. You are always within your rights to ask whether your doctor has washed his hands before meeting you and how your instruments were cleaned. This is not a typical way Valley Fever is transmitted. However, *Coccidioides* is already serious and you should not have to deal with the added worry of being infected with another organism in the doctor's office or hospital.

There is no reason for your doctors ever to be upset by being asked whether their hands are clean, as the Centers for Disease Control have been promoting an ongoing campaign for years to prevent doctors from spreading infections through poor hand hygiene.[42] The CDC even established a web site for their Guidelines for Hand Hygiene in Healthcare Settings:
http://www.cdc.gov/handhygiene/

If an infection from your doctor's hands isn't enough to worry about, it has been noted that a doctor's tie could also harbor infectious organisms. Neckties are not as frequently washed as hands or other clothing items, and often drape where they can touch patients. Even if patients are not touched by a necktie, "it might not occur to doctors to wash their hands after handling their ties" and this problem might apply to many personal items. "Other research has found that doctors' pens, cellphones and pagers can harbor potentially harmful micro-organisms."[191]

Ask About the Lab Facilities

Find out where your blood tests are being sent. If your Complement Fixation titers are being tracked in the hope they will indicate how well your doctor's treatments are working, and the tests are being conducted at different laboratories, this could be a problem. Different labs may use different materials and procedures, making the results of the tests inconsistent. This inconsistency may make it difficult or impossible for doctors to find a meaningful correlation between your titer's results and the severity of your Valley Fever.[215]

Beware of Drug Interactions

Be certain your doctor is aware of any medications you are taking and how they might interact with any drugs or treatments that might be considered for Valley Fever.

Keep a Critical Eye on Your Prescription

If you are given a prescription, ask exactly what your drug will look like, how many pills should be in each bottle, and the prescribed dose of each pill. Then when the prescription is filled, check the label to make sure it says you have received the correct drug at the correct quantity and the correct dose per pill. Inside the bottle, if the color is different, or if it's not what you expected, don't assume that the company just changed its shape or color. Ask the pharmacist if it is correct and ask your doctor as well. If there is any error, be cautious because other errors may be present. Double checking could save your life from the wrong drugs.

Take Charge

Some doctors who have a medical ignorance of this disease refuse to test for Valley Fever because they are "sure" it couldn't cause certain symptoms, even when medical documentation proves otherwise. Remember that you are the one paying the medical professionals, and that it is their job to listen to *you*. If your current doctor refuses to test for this disease and you want a test, find a doctor who will cooperate. A patient whose concerns are ignored is unlikely to be treated well, even in cases that are totally unrelated to Valley Fever.

Other doctors refuse to treat cocci even when it is diagnosed because they focus on risk factors for *severe* Valley Fever. These doctors ignore the fact that anyone can have a severe, chronic, or fatal case no matter how mild their symptoms may appear at one time and regardless as to whether they fit into a high risk group.

Patients who repeatedly had Valley Fever symptoms and positive tests had even reported that their doctors said these tests *must be wrong*, even though their cases perfectly matched Valley Fever's incubation period and symptoms. Some patients whose tests were positive for years had doctors erroneously tell them another disease must be the cause of their ongoing symptoms since Valley Fever "wouldn't last this long." Surprisingly, some of these patients had even received these erroneous opinions from doctors who are highly regarded as medical experts. You must find a doctor who is willing to take your concerns and this disease seriously.

Reluctance to Diagnose Valley Fever

Via e-mail we are sometimes asked "what happens when I still feel sick and the doctor doesn't want to accept the low titer and symptoms as a sign of ongoing Valley Fever?" This happens frequently when the patient's symptoms continue while there is a low titer like 1:2 or when recent VF tests come up negative.

This is a common concern we have read in our Valley Fever Survivor questionnaires and e-mails. From my experience, the answer could be that the doctor...

A) tries more tests, perhaps for Valley Fever again or for other diseases.

B) listens to the patient's symptoms, considers that VF is still there, and goes on a hunch that Valley Fever may still be active. This leads to "empirical treatment" (a guess) with antifungal drugs.

C) sees the low or negative titer, has a hunch that VF is *not* causing whatever symptoms are present, and decides to treat another illness empirically.

D) sees the low or negative titer, has a hunch that VF is *not* causing whatever symptoms are present, and sends the patient to a psychiatrist or a psychologist. The doctor believes the ongoing symptoms are all in the patient's mind.

E) says "Did you know that Valley Fever is a benign disease? Your symptoms will go away on their own" and ignores patients who complain of ongoing VF symptoms.

Although there are many illnesses that can harm people whether or not they have been infected with Valley Fever, that is no excuse to disregard the disease altogether. Regrettably, some doctors' minds seem to shut down when faced with complicated cases of Valley Fever. Perhaps this ignorant and often demeaning attitude is why Arizona released $50,000 in emergency funding to train doctors during the state's record breaking Valley Fever epidemic in 2006. Patients need to become their own advocates and should seek medical attention elsewhere if they are dissatisfied with their current care.

Frustration with Misdiagnosis and Medical Care

Theresa is a patient who contacted us about her very frustrating medical ordeal. When it comes to her horrible level of medical mistreatment, she is far from alone. There have been many others with Valley Fever who described just as many hassles with doctors that refused to believe the disease could cause a problem. Unfortunately, many of these people had suffered without an accurate diagnosis over the course of years rather than months.

We hope that many doctors and nurses will read Theresa's story as well so they can learn from the mistakes of others.

Theresa Dyson
Diagnosed with VF at age 35
Tucson, AZ

Before my Valley Fever, I was a healthy 35 year old living in Tucson, Arizona. I have been living here for twelve years and have five children. I don't work outside, just the typical yard work and swimming. But I do live near construction. Who doesn't in Tucson?

I have also been suffering from extreme back, neck and joint pain for at least 6 years. I have been to my primary physician, chiropractors and shrinks only to be told I have depression or that I am just too stressed out. In other words, it's all in my head. I have been on anti-depressants, anti-anxiety medication, popped more Tylenol and Advil than I can remember, and still no relief.

Within the last six months my symptoms have become unbearable, accompanied by a horrible nagging cough, bodyaches, headache, fever, chills, lethargy and light sensitivity. My primary doctor ordered a MRI and a CAT scan. They called me with the results only to say I was fine. So after a face to face visit with my primary doctor, he decided that I am depressed and puts me on a cocktail of Lamictal, a bipolar depression medicine, which caused a severe reaction (my throat closing up, worse body aches.)

Several calls later, I finally convinced my Dr. that I needed to get off of it. He then puts me on high doses of Zoloft and Wellbutrin. These medicines have done nothing for my symptoms. So several doctor visits and co-pays later, my doctor orders full metabolic labs with a test for rheumatoid arthritis!

After not hearing from the nurse on my results, I contact the doctor only to be told that "Your labs are perfect!" and "I will refer you to a psychiatrist and physical therapist." I couldn't believe it. He also said that he needed me to come in again for a "med" check for the anti-depressants. Well, I declined to contact the psychiatrist and physical therapist and reluctantly made another appointment with my primary care doctor.

At the appointment he said I should be feeling so much better because of the meds. I told him that I would feel better if my hacking cough, fever, body aches etc. would go away. He said I had the flu and just to go home and wait it out. Leaving his office in complete and utter frustration, I just broke down and cried and slept and cried and slept. Feeling worse and defeated, I decided to take matters in my own hands, and turn on the computer and do a little research of my symptoms. Voilà!

I found your site and it all started to make sense to me. Immediately, I call my doctor and asked for a Valley Fever test. His nurse responded with a "Well I'll have to ask the doctor, but I don't think that is what you have!" [eds: What right did that nurse have to make that statement?]

A week later I get a call back from her telling me she had an order at their front office for the blood test. The very next morning I pulled my tired, achy body out of bed and went to get the test. I was sure I had it. I was actually looking forward to the call confirming that they found out what was wrong with me. Instead, on Halloween this year, as I'm painfully volunteering in my daughter's classroom, I get a call from a random nurse saying "Your test came back, and there is nothing wrong with you. Your blood is perfect."

"WHAT?" I asked. You're saying nothing is wrong?"

"Yes," she said, "you are fine." In utter frustration and in respect for my daughter and her classmates, I hung up the phone. Needless to say, I went home that day, took my usual cocktail of ant-depressants, Advil and Motrin, and cried myself to sleep.

A week to the day later, Nov 7th 2007, at 7am I got a call from the first nurse who reluctantly ordered the VF test, and she says, "Theresa you have Valley Fever. Your test came back positive and we need you here next week."

Filled with relief and fear I say, "I knew it. What is my titer level? And who called me last week and said I was fine?"

She says, "I don't know what you're talking about and your test just came back positive and we need to see you." So I made the appointment for next week, Nov 13 at 10am. Then I immediately went back on your web site and read everything I could. I have learned so much!

Although I feel that I have just started a long journey, I want to thank you for leading me in the right direction. I have so many questions, fears, and anger. Where do I start? I have 5 kids that need so much attention. I have been too ill to keep up with them lately and I feel an enormous guilt and anger for that. I don't want to continue to miss out on their lives because I feel so terrible. I also have a very hardworking husband who needs me to work to help support our family. I'm in no condition to work! What do people in my situation do?

She provided more information after we had contacted her.

Well I wish I had good news to tell you about how my doctor helped me with my situation, but I don't. I went to the Nov. 13th appointment, waited over an hour to see him only to be told, yes, you have Valley Fever. I asked him what my titer level was and he said he didn't know, but he showed me the "positive" result on the lab.

Then I asked him, "what next?" He said he would order a chest x-ray and that I can go that very day. So I went to a radiology clinic and got the x-ray that very day. Would you believe that I have called and left several messages for the doctor only to get a call back on the 20th from his nurse asking why I haven't gotten the x-ray?! I told her where I went and she said that she called the wrong clinic.

I told her that I have called at least four times and that I would appreciate a call back right away with the results. She never called me back! I have called twice since and still haven't heard back. So up until I received your email, I have all but just given up! I still feel sick and tired and achy. I have never in my life dealt with anything like this before! I refuse to go in again and pay another co-pay. I will look through the phone book today for a pulmonary or infectious disease doctor.

I first found out what Valley Fever was when my dog was acting very tired and sick. I took him to the vet and learned that he had Valley Fever. They put him on meds, and did very well on them, so they took him off. I thought that only dogs could get the disease until I found your website by typing in "Valley Fever."

It is not a rare event for us to receive stories like this. In fact, stories like Theresa's are common and stories with a timely and accurate diagnosis are an infrequent exception rather than the rule.

> What do experts consider the right way to treat Valley Fever cases? A good indication may be the guidelines provided by the Infectious Disease Society of America (IDSA).[98] Read the guidelines at the web address below:
> http://www.journals.uchicago.edu/doi/full/10.1086/496991

A Personal Message from Sharon

We at valleyfeversurvivor.com are truly sorry that you have been infected with this incurable disease. It is important for you to understand that you must be your own advocate when it comes to your medical care. It would be a good idea to take someone with you for your doctor appointments. When you are feeling so ill it is impossible to remember everything the doctor tells you or to ask all the right questions. Before going to your appointment, make a list of all your questions so that either you or the individual attending the appointment with you can ask them.

Some people may tell you they had Valley Fever and it was like a simple cold, but do not let anyone minimize the symptoms you experience. It is important to realize that you have contracted a serious disease and your well being spiritually, mentally, physically and emotionally may be compromised. Your life may be completely turned upside down and you don't know what to expect now or for the future. Please know that it is okay to be confused, upset, and even angry. That is only natural.

Many people suffering with Valley Fever look perfectly healthy on the outside. This is a major reason family, friends, co-workers, and even many doctors don't understand how you could possibly be so sick on the inside.

Not everyone in your family will understand or even accept what is happening to you but it is very important for you to realize that you matter and need to do what is best for your health. This can be very difficult when your health is at risk.

Know that it is important for you to rest, rest, and rest. Fatigue is a major part of the disease. You may feel out of control but listening to your body, following the doctors' orders, and getting the rest that you need at this time will help to bring perspective and control back into your life.

Learn to prioritize what is really necessary and those things you can let go of. Try not to put pressure on yourself unnecessarily. If you have financial issues, you may need to apply for social security or even your state's disability. Sometimes it may just be workmen's compensation.

You may need to hire someone or get a friend to help with daily chores. It always feels better to have your surroundings as normal as possible. Most importantly, take care of yourself. Regardless of your life's previous circumstances, you have now been put in the position where you must come first.

The Valley Fever community at valleyfeversurvivor.com is a very caring and loving place to be. If you would like to talk with other people who have Valley Fever, feel free to join the Valley Fever Survivor Message Board at the web site:

http://www.valleyfeversurvivor.com/vfsmb

It has been extremely helpful to our readers and in some cases is the only place they can go to get the support they need. If you ever need anyone to talk with we are a click away.

Dave and I send our love and prayers for recovery to everyone with Valley Fever and their loved ones. We hope our work can provide people with the help and courage they need to deal with this illness.

Sharon

Testing and Diagnosis

At a Glance

- Blood and cerebrospinal fluid tests for Valley Fever do not find the fungus itself, but rather antibodies to *Coccidioides* spp. spores.
- There are many chemical procedures to find these antibodies. Some tests have a titer—a number that may be helpful to track the severity of the case. A titer of 1:16 or higher is serious and means it is likely that the fungus had spread (disseminated) from the patient's lung to other areas of the body.
- Valley Fever tests may fail to find antibodies even when the patient has the disease.
- X-rays, MRIs and other imaging procedures can find lesions that are commonly misdiagnosed as cancer but may actually be caused by Valley Fever.
- Biopsies of lesions and damaged tissue can find the fungus directly. Positive biopsies are absolute proof of a *Coccidioides* infection.
- Bronchoscopies and other medical procedures can take fluids and biopsies from patients to recover the fungus and diagnose Valley Fever.

The Importance of a Valley Fever Diagnosis

Since fungal diseases have so little public mindshare, patients and doctors alike tend to assume bacteria or viruses are responsible for undiagnosed illnesses. Many of valleyfeversurvivor.com's questionnaire respondents can attest to the fact that bacterial antibiotics have been given to them empirically.

Empirical treatments are drugs given to a patient based on a doctor's guess about what might help when the illness' cause has not been proven. A great deal of harm can be caused when people are given the wrong drugs. Furthermore, it is extraordinarily rare among our e-mail contacts and questionnaire respondents ever to receive antifungal drugs empirically. This suggests that a laboratory diagnosis is the only way patients in need of Valley Fever treatment are ever likely to receive the proper medication. Even in the heart of the endemic regions it often seems like doctors only consider Valley Fever as a last resort if they consider it at all.

Understanding Antibody Tests for Valley Fever

The most common way Valley Fever is diagnosed is by studying the immune response of patients. Often this occurs in serology, the study of serum (the part of the blood that contains antibodies). Cerebrospinal fluid (CSF) taken from a lumbar puncture can also be used to test for an immune response. Lumbar punctures are also known as spinal taps.

For many diseases, antibodies are created by the immune system to assist white blood cells in the body's defense against a specific invading organism. Although antibodies are typically produced during a Valley Fever infection, they are unfortunately ineffective when fighting Valley Fever,[215] leaving the immune system's work to white blood cells (such as CD4+ T lymphocytes) instead.[127] However, the fact that antibodies are specific to *Coccidioides* and easier to detect than the fungus itself makes them important for the disease's diagnosis.

> Infections are often compared to an invading army. When the war metaphor is applied to Valley Fever, white blood cells are the defending army and antibodies are signal flares that indicate the presence of invading *Coccidioides* spores to the doctors.

To find the antibodies, antigens are used. An antigen is a foreign substance that the immune system reacts to in a specific way. For example, parts of *Coccidioides* fungi stimulate the immune system to produce antibodies, and the antibodies react to these antigens. It is possible to put antigens into a sample of a patient's blood serum (or cerebrospinal fluid) and to see whether there is a reaction or what kind of reaction there is.

A positive reaction means the patient has Valley Fever. The types of antibodies found in Valley Fever tests are either Immunoglobulin M (IgM) antibodies (commonly found early in active infections and sometimes they persist) or Immunoglobulin G (IgG) antibodies. IgG antibodies tend to appear later in an infection, sometimes as the case improves or even when it does not. IgG antibodies are useful to show that there is an ongoing infection or a previous infection.[12]

When the antibody tests show a strong reaction to the antigen, they are considered positive. Tests with a minimal reaction are considered negative, although there are many instances of Valley Fever patients with negative tests whose infections were proven after biopsies or autopsies. Such failures of the test to detect the antibodies are known as false negatives.

The manufacturers of laboratory tests often recommend that these tests are given three or more weeks apart to account for the immune system's sometimes delayed reaction to Valley Fever.

Even then, there are possibilities for false negatives. 30% of patients known to have chronic lung disease from Valley Fever do not have positive antibody tests. Also, 10% of cerebrospinal fluid tests may be negative even in people who have meningitis from Valley Fever.[12] Some data suggests an even higher percentage of false negatives may occur.

In a 2006 study of people known to be infected with Valley Fever, false negatives occurred in 18% of EIA tests, 29% of immunodiffusion tests, and 44% of compliment fixation titer tests.[202]

Some of our questionnaire respondents report that they were only given one Valley Fever test (with a false negative at first) and had to go on for months while told their symptoms were not from Valley Fever. As their disease worsened, they were either given another test or their Valley Fever was diagnosed later through a biopsy. Other patients who were ultimately proven to have Valley Fever had not been given a Valley Fever test for years because doctors did not believe Valley Fever could cause their symptoms. False negative test results only worsen the diagnosis problem.

"[S]erologic tests alone cannot rule out the disease."[215]

There can also be a reaction between the antigens for Valley Fever and antibodies for some other fungal diseases, leading to a false positive result. False positives for Valley Fever are rare. They occur when the patient is infected with other systemic fungal diseases like histoplasmosis or blastomycosis.[147]

> Medical literature only occasionally mentions false positives. In the thousands of questionnaires and survey responses we received, there was only one false positive Valley Fever diagnosis. In that case, the patient's disease was actually histoplasmosis. In our other responses and the medical literature, there were many false negatives.

Some doctors we have interviewed considered the UC Davis laboratory to be the "gold standard" for excellence in *Coccidioides* testing, with the implication that tests sent elsewhere might have less credible results. If testing specimens are not kept sealed and at the proper temperature, and sometimes even if the testing material is not stored or transported properly, there can be lab errors that result in false negatives.

Due to potential laboratory or storage errors, where the blood test is evaluated (and by whom) can make the difference between a positive or negative result. This is even true with biopsies and cultures, the forms of testing that do not specifically search for antibodies.

Another issue of increasing concern is that testing and patient documentation may not necessarily be sent to the best laboratories, but instead to cheap outsourcing partners that are selected "based on contractual agreements with outsource providers. This leads to confusion and frustration for the doctor and patient alike, and occasionally, to medical error."[45] Although treatment is far from perfect, errors in Valley Fever's diagnosis can be very costly to patients' health and lives.

Immune System Issues

Sometimes Valley Fever patients will not have positive complement fixation titers or enzyme immunoassays. While the tests might even have been performed to perfection with perfect specimens, sometimes the body does not react to the fungus. It frequently takes two weeks after symptoms begin before the early antibodies (IgM) are introduced into the bloodstream.[32] The IgM response is also likely to fade within four[44] to six months,[16] making the level of IgG antibodies more critical for doctors to follow.

A test that would only check for one type of antibody to Valley Fever could ignore the other type, thereby missing the diagnosis.

Antibodies may also be undetectable in patients with immune system impairments. Immune system problems could be obvious like AIDS or malnutrition, or perhaps be conditions that patients may not expect like organ transplantation, diabetes, corticosteroid use, and simple stress.

Complement Fixation Titers

A complement fixation (CF) titer is a common test for *Coccidioides* antibodies in blood serum or cerebrospinal fluid (CSF). In an example with serum from a blood test, it "is diluted with an equal amount of salt solution and tested for valley fever. The serum is diluted more and more (one part serum to 2, 4, 8, 16, 32, 64, 128, 256, etc. parts of salt water) and tested at each dilution until a positive test for valley fever can no longer be detected."[67]

Therefore, if no antibodies are detected when the serum is diluted with two parts salt solution, it is considered a titer of <1:2. This is read as "less than one to two" or "below one to two." The test is then considered negative for Valley Fever.

If antibodies are found at that level the test is considered positive, and the current mixture is diluted further by doubling the amount of salt solution again.

A measurement of "1:4" would be read as "one to four" and means antibodies were visible when one part of the test fluid was serum and four parts were solution, but would not be positive when more solution was added. "1:8" would be read as "one to eight" and it means the test was positive for antibodies when the liquid tested was one part serum and eight parts solution, but not when more solution was added to that mixture.

The test procedure is to keep diluting the serum by doubling and redoubling the salt solution, so the next titers are 1:16, 1:32, 1:64 and so on. An extraordinarily high titer of 1:2048 is rare but still occurs from time to time.

The higher the second number, the more antibodies there were and the more severe the illness often has been. For decades, doctors have known that a titer of 1:2 is considered low and titers that are at[236] 1:16 or higher[233] have been considered serious and likely to indicate dissemination in humans. Doctors have considered titers of 1:8 serious, but not necessarily likely to indicate dissemination. High titers in animals have not been as predictive of dissemination as high titers in people.

If more than one test were taken over the course of a few weeks or months, rising titers would indicate that the disease may be worsening and may need stronger antifungal therapy. Decreasing titers can indicate that the patient is getting better, and that the current course of treatment may be working. Doctors must evaluate their patients' symptoms and cannot trust the trend in CF titer tests completely. The connection between a titer and the severity of a patient's Valley Fever is not absolute.

Complement fixation titers famously test for IgG[200] but can evaluate both IgM and IgG antibodies.[12] When doctors see the IgM rise early in the case, only to fall while IgG antibodies remain, that is fairly typical in Valley Fever patients. IgM antibodies typically disappear in four months.[44] IgG antibodies can be used to track the effectiveness of antifungal treatment over longer periods of time since decreasing symptoms with decreasing IgG titers usually suggest therapy is working.[32]

Sometimes the IgG titers might not be reduced to <1:2 by the time antifungal therapy is scheduled to end. When this happens, doctors may choose to have their patients take antifungal drugs for a longer period of time, sometimes at a lower dose.

Other Antibody Tests

Other antibody tests are available. These include tube precipitin tests, immunodiffusion, enzyme immunoassays (also known as EIA), and the category of enzyme immunoassays known as ELISA tests (ELISA stands for "enzyme linked immunosorbent assay").

These procedures can tell whether a patient is infected with Valley Fever because they can find antibodies to *Coccidioides*, but most of them cannot tell anything about the severity of the Valley Fever infection in the patient. The layman's description of the procedure involved in these tests is that a part of the patient's serum is placed with specific chemicals to see if a chemical reaction with the antibodies happens.

Like the complement fixation titer, these can also have false negatives and occasional false positives if the patient has antibodies to a different systemic fungal infection.

Many tests for Valley Fever are only *qualitative*, meaning they are intended to find a positive or negative response specifically for Valley Fever and not for any other disease. Qualitative tests will only be positive or negative. The complement fixation titer is useful because it is also *quantitative*, meaning it indicates how serious the antibody response is to Valley Fever. However, this does not necessarily make all other tests less useful.

There are both qualitative and quantitative immunodiffusion tests, although the qualitative immunodiffusion tests are more common. ELISA tests are qualitative only. Latex agglutination tests check for IgM antibodies and are qualitative as well, and they are sometimes combined with immunodiffusion tests to find IgG antibodies.[135]

Along with the complement fixation titers, the most commonly used tests are ELISA (which can check for IgM and IgG antibodies), and immunodiffusion (which is typically used for IgM antibodies and sometimes IgG). A titer checking the IgG antibodies from a quantitative immunodiffusion test is expected to have similar results to the complement fixation titer test.[200]

For patients who want to understand the lab results of their blood tests, they will notice a test that says "*Coccidioides* antibody," the name of the test, and a number. The number is the result of the test. Often on that same page will be a number next to the words "reference interval" or "reference values." These numbers show how the test is supposed to be read, which numbers are negative (meaning they did not find evidence of the disease), which are positive (to indicate the patient has Valley Fever), and which might indicate an inconclusive test.

Although the immunodiffusion test results and complement fixation test results can be reported in two to four days, ELISA tests may take one to five days for results.[13, 14]

ELISA Tests

0.9 or less (read as "zero point nine" to indicate it is below "one") in the IgM part of an ELISA test means no IgM antibodies were detected. Anything in that range is a negative test. Sometimes a value in the negative range is said to be within the "reference interval."

The range of 1.0 to 1.4 is questionable for the antibodies, so there may or may not be an IgM response and another test might be useful in 10-14 days to see if there is a change. The words "indeterminate" or "equivocal" are often used in that range of uncertain diagnosis.

A reaction of 1.5 or higher indicates a positive test for the antibodies. The IgG response in an ELISA test is likely to be a different number from the IgM value, and the IgG's number would also be interpreted as negative if it were 0.9 or less, positive if it were at 1.5 or higher, and questionable in between.[12,156]

Many other labs have *Coccidioides* ELISA tests that lead to the same numbers as above for negative, uncertain, and positive results. However, some labs[249] considered their ELISA *Coccidioides* antibody test to be positive above 1.1 rather than 1.4.

EIA Tests

The Enzyme Immunoassay Test (EIA) is negative with test values below 0.150, indeterminate from 0.150 to 0.199, and positive at 0.200 and above.[115]

As with the ELISA test, some EIA tests may utilize different numbers for results. Another brand's EIA test is negative below 1.0, positive at or above 1.5, and indeterminate between those numbers.[136]

Immunodiffusion Tests

A qualitative immunodiffusion test will either show positive or negative. It primarily detects the IgM antibodies that appear earliest in a Valley Fever case but the "IgG antibod[ies] may also be demonstrated" in a part of the test's reaction.[16]

Patients "who have leaky blood-brain barriers" might have antibodies from the blood in their cerebrospinal fluid. While this is not common, if such a patient has a qualitative immunodiffusion test to check for antibodies in the cerebrospinal fluid (a telltale sign of meningitis), it could pose a problem: If the patient is suffering from a Valley Fever case that does *not* have meningitis, the cerebrospinal fluid may test positive and wrongly indicate meningitis.[200]

Tube Precipitin

A tube precipitin titer is either positive or negative. It would find the IgM antibodies, so this test might help primarily in the first months of the illness' diagnosis.[12]

Latex Agglutination

Latex agglutination tests specifically bind to IgM antibodies so they can be identified, although labs can sell these tests paired with an immunodiffusion "IDCF" test to identify IgG antibodies too. Both of these tests would be qualitative and, therefore, only indicate a positive or negative response to *Coccidioides* antibodies but not the severity of the illness. The latex agglutination portion of the test takes only a little more than ten minutes for results and the IDCF test it is paired with takes 24 hours for results. The IDCF test could take over 48 hours longer when trying to confirm a negative result.

False positives from latex agglutination might occur when rheumatoid factor (an antibody often found in arthritis patients) is present.[135] That can be a problem since Valley Fever has been nicknamed "Desert Rheumatism" for the rheumatoid arthritis it can cause.

Lab Lingo

When reading laboratory result documents, they may use some unfamiliar symbols. It is handy to know the difference between < and >. The one pointing to the left means "less than" and the symbol pointing to the right means "greater than." As with the complement fixation titer, a reading of <1 is read as "less than one."

Further, the name of the antibodies tested should appear on the test. Sometimes a test for IgM antibodies will be written with TP to indicate the tube precipitin test and sometimes the IgG antibodies will be found with the CF since they are commonly found with Complement Fixation titers. Immunodiffusion tests sometimes have the titer for each antibody written as IDTP and IDCF to show the test for IgM and IgG antibodies, respectively.

Sometimes the antibodies are simply named as IgM or IgG.

"IgG," "CF," "IDCF" and "Complement fixing antibodies" might all refer to the same type of antibodies in a Valley Fever test or when reading medical documents.

Likewise "latex agglutinating," "LA," "TP," and "IDTP" all could refer to the IgM antibodies.

Here is an example of how to read your own test. If you only found a negative test for IgM antibodies on your personal testing paperwork and it had been a year after your primary symptoms began, this might be expected since IgM antibodies tend to wane over time as the IgG antibodies increase in number.

IgG antibodies are usually the longest lasting, and they indicate how well a Valley Fever case is progressing over the medium to long term.

Depending on how early the test was taken, it is possible that IgM might be the only antibody response, rendering an IgG test useless. If the test is taken too soon in the course of a patient's Valley Fever (usually the first month) or the antibodies are not being produced, both antibody types would be negative. Also, years after the initial infection, there might be no titer at all, even when people have ongoing symptoms.

> When reading the lab report from any test, it is good to check for the terms "reference interval," "negative," "positive," "indeterminate," and "equivocal" so you can understand exactly what the results will mean, no matter which lab handled your test.

A Quick Review:

- IgM antibodies are the earliest antibodies found for Valley Fever. They usually appear after the first month of infection and disappear a few months later. They often indicate an early or ongoing infection.

- IgG antibodies are found weeks or months after IgM antibody production begins in a Valley Fever infection. They often indicate an ongoing infection or one that had occurred previously and may or may not be causing symptoms. These antibodies last the longest.

- Complement Fixation Titer tests check for both IgM and IgG antibodies. A <1:2 response is negative, 1:8 or higher tends to be serious and titers of 1:16 or over usually indicate disseminated infection. The higher the number after the colon, the more severe the case tends to be. It takes 2-4 days for lab results. Complement Fixation Titer tests for IgG antibodies can be used to track the effectiveness of antifungal treatment or the severity of the illness, since decreasing symptoms and titers usually suggest therapy is working.

- ELISA and EIA tests check for both IgM and IgG antibodies, although they are qualitative so they cannot describe the severity of the disease. Different labs will have different values for positive, negative, and equivocal (uncertain) results. It takes 1-5 days for results.

- Qualitative immunodiffusion tests check for both IgM and IgG antibodies. The result will be either positive or negative without a descriptive number. A quantitative immunodiffusion test for IgG antibodies (IDCF) could have results that indicate the severity of the illness or the usefulness of the therapy, very much like the complement fixation titer tests would.[200] It takes 2-4 days to obtain results.

- Tube Precipitin and Latex Agglutination tests evaluate the presence of IgM only. The test will be either positive or negative without a descriptive number. Since the IgM antibodies appear earliest in a Valley Fever infection, these tests are likely to be most useful near the start of patients' symptoms.

- Latex agglutination tests for IgM but can be used in combination with an immunodiffusion IgG test. The result can either be negative (symbolized with the dash character "-") or positive, although the 1+ to 4+ rating does not necessarily correlate with disease severity. This test takes over two days for results.

Quick Facts About Antibody Tests

- 30% of patients known to have chronic lung disease from Valley Fever do not have positive antibody tests.
- 10% of cerebrospinal fluid tests may be negative even in people who have meningitis from Valley Fever.
- Antibodies may be undetectable in patients with compromised immune systems.
- False negatives can occur. If stored samples and cultures are improperly handled or transported, positive samples can become unreadable.
- If more than one quantitative test is taken over the course of a few weeks (CF titer or quantitative immunodiffusion), rising titers would indicate that the disease may be worsening and may need stronger antifungal therapy.
- Antibody tests are not always accurate. A 2006 study evaluated many serologic tests in people known to have Valley Fever due to positive cultures. The study found that the EIA tests were positive 82% of the time, immunodiffusion tests were positive 71% of the time, and complement fixation titers were positive only 56% of the time. The timing of testing in the course of a patient's illness can make a difference in the tests' accuracy. Although that data was not available to fully explain these numbers, these statistics clearly indicate the need to consider Valley Fever as a possibility even after one or more negative antibody tests.[202]

Other Methods of Diagnosis for Valley Fever

- Biopsies of lesions or some bodily tissues could be cultured for *Coccidioides*. Surgical, shave, or needle biopsies all can be used.
- Sputum or urine samples may be used to detect *Coccidioides*. Urine samples have rarely helped to diagnose patients.
- Bronchoscopies remove samples from the lung for culture.
- Imaging tests (x-rays, CT scans, MRIs, and bone scans) and other blood tests also can help with diagnosis.

Biopsies, Samples, and Cultures

When Valley Fever causes lesions on a patient's skin or organs, and sometimes when it inflames tissue like synovial joints (causing arthritis), a culture may diagnose the disease. Cultures are the laboratory growth of organisms from a sample of bodily material from the patient.

A biopsy is a removal of a lesion or some bodily tissue to help in diagnosis, and the typical way to culture *Coccidioides* from a person is to use the biopsied tissue. This tissue is called a sample.

Biopsies can be surgical, meaning that doctors cut directly into the patient to remove part of a lesion or tissue.

Shave biopsies are also possible, where thin slices of sample tissue can be cut off of easily accessible lesions, as if "shaving" the top of the lesion.

Needle biopsies work by inserting a medical syringe into a lesion, pulling back on the plunger to vacuum material into the syringe, and then removing the needle. On a pus filled skin lesion, this is fairly easy. When a lung lesion needs to be biopsied, sometimes the procedure is called a "fine needle biopsy," emphasizing the thinness of the syringe needle used for the delicate procedure.

While there is some risk of deflating the lung with needle biopsies of lung lesions, Valley Fever's lung lesions are frequently misdiagnosed as cancer. This misdiagnosis is fairly dangerous, since cancer often requires lung resection surgery, while Valley Fever lung lesions may not require surgery at all. Having all or part of one's lung removed is bad enough, but if the surgery is unnecessary that is a terrible mistake. Biopsies could potentially save the patients from unnecessary surgery when they are falsely diagnosed with cancer but find out too late that they have Valley Fever instead.

Samples can also be taken without a biopsy. They could come from sputum (spit) or occasionally urine, although the latter has rarely helped to diagnose patients. Even when a patient is able to spit freely, "steam-induced sputum has a better yield" for diagnostic purposes. To simplify testing further, sometimes there is no need even to culture the sample if the biopsied sample is examined under a microscope and *Coccidioides* spores are seen. Although it tends not to be as effective as other tests, this is still worthwhile because it is considered quick, cheap, and easy.[241] The spherules and endospores produced by *Coccidioides* spp. should raise suspicion of Valley Fever when identified visually.

Material for culture or microscope viewing can also be taken by a bronchoscopy. This medical procedure involves a long flexible probe (a bronchoscope) that physicians put through the patient's nose or mouth, down the throat, and into the lung. The doctor can use the bronchoscope to see inside the patient's lung and take a biopsy or sample of fluid. Sometimes there will also be a "bronchial wash" where the bronchoscope sprays saline fluid within the lung to make the collection of fluid easier.

Depending on the anesthesia or the doctor's technique, a bronchoscopy can be either an uneventful or incredibly painful test. Even more complicated ways of getting biopsies directly from the lung include the mediastinoscope, which is inserted through a surgical incision above the sternum, and the thoracoscope, put through an incision in the chest.[67] Fortunately none of our Valley Fever Survivor questionnaire respondents reported that they were required to have either of these two surgical procedures just for a test.

Testing a Cultured Specimen

It may take two to three weeks to culture (grow) a *Coccidioides* specimen,[71] although enough may be grown to be identified in as few as four days.[215] A DNA probe is performed after the specimen has been cultured. The DNA probe reacts with cultured samples to see whether *Coccidioides* is present. Results can be reported in less than 24 hours from that time.[15] However, the DNA probe is fast enough that a cultured mold can be confirmed to be *Coccidioides* in a lab in less than three hours.[241]

As with antibody tests, improperly handled or stored samples and cultures can make a positive sample unreadable in the lab so it becomes a false negative.

Skin Tests

Decades ago, there were skin tests for Valley Fever using reagents called coccidioidin and spherulin. Although they were made differently, both tests were conducted by scratching the skin with a slight injection of non-infectious *Coccidioides* material and then checking for an immune response on the skin 24 and then 48 hours later. This test would quickly determine if someone had a previous infection.

This made skin tests useful for epidemiologists (professionals who study the causes and prevalence of disease). Since both tests are now unavailable for commercial use and the new version of the spherulin test has not yet been released, it is unlikely that skin tests would be used to diagnose Valley Fever cases at present. The skin test also does not work during the first few weeks of a patient's Valley Fever infection, making it unlikely that it would be used for clinical diagnoses in the future.

Supplemental Testing

Neither an erythrocyte sedimentation rate test nor an eosinophil count test can diagnose Valley Fever or a specific disease. Imaging tests are only able to reveal the damage to the body, but cannot prove whether Valley Fever or another disease caused the damage. However, even without a certain diagnosis, all of these tests may provide valuable clues that Valley Fever might be active.

Imaging Tests

Imaging tests like x-rays, CT scans, MRIs, bone scans, PET scans and others frequently help in the diagnosis of Valley Fever. If a patient's symptoms began within 1-4 weeks of travel or residence in an endemic area, and a lesion is found by an imaging scan, then this may be a tip-off to a doctor that the lesion could have been caused by Valley Fever. Lesions have also been found later in Valley Fever cases.

Although many Valley Fever patients are first diagnosed because of a suspicious chest x-ray or CT scan, there are hidden dangers to these imaging tests. They are outlined in the "What You Need to Know Before You See A Doctor" Chapter's section titled "Risks Associated with Some Tests and Treatments."

Erythrocyte Sedimentation Rate Tests

Erythrocyte sedimentation is a test to see how rapidly red blood cells settle when in a specific controlled condition. This test is often performed to check for inflammation in a variety of diseases.

Although tests for erythrocyte sedimentation are not commonly used for Valley Fever, a study found that an erythrocyte sedimentation rate over 15mm/hr (millimeters per hour) correlated with dissemination in 96% of the disseminated Valley Fever cases examined. "The level of erythrocyte sedimentation rate elevation may be added to the list of predictors for disseminated disease."[64]

Eosinophil Count Tests

Eosinophilia, an increase in the white blood cells called eosinophils, also can be a clue for the presence of Valley Fever.[64] After a 32-year old Japanese man went on a vacation to Arizona to play golf, he returned home and was coughing up blood one month later. Although the Japanese physicians noticed his eosinophilia, lung cavities, and nodules, they misdiagnosed his case as tuberculosis, having him take several unneeded tuberculosis drugs over the course of three months. Only as things got worse and a biopsy was taken was he ultimately diagnosed with Valley Fever. "Eosinophilia was closely related to the severity of the disease" so it can be another clue for wary doctors to consider.[184]

A pleural effusion is liquid, usually blood or lymph, that is released into the membrane around the lungs as a part of many different illnesses. This fluid can be tested in a procedure called a pleural fluid analysis, which can find eosinophils. "Pleural effusions are common in hospitalized patients with Coccidioidomycosis. Pleural fluid eosinophilia should alert [the] clinician to *Coccidioides*" since this organism may be the cause.[178]

Drugs and Treatment

At a Glance

- Lesions and inflammation caused by Valley Fever may be treated with surgery.
- The antifungal drugs that treat Valley Fever have many side effects that can be as bad as the disease. Higher doses of these drugs increase the likelihood and severity of these side effects more than lower doses would, but higher doses may also increase the drugs' effectiveness against Valley Fever.
- Amphotericin B is a powerful, decades-old Valley Fever medication. It can be put directly in the spinal fluid and has typically been reserved for the most severe cases. It typically has the most severe side effects.
- Azole drugs like Diflucan (fluconazole), Sporanox (itraconazole), and Vfend (voriconazole) are more typical treatments.
- The combination of drugs for Valley Fever with drugs for other conditions may produce terrible side effects.
- You can keep up with the latest drug information on the web.
- Relapse rates are as high as 75% only one year after stopping therapy.
- Organizations offer free or lower cost for medications if you qualify. One organization even provides medical assistance for pets.

Surgery

Lesions are bodily tissue altered due to a state of illness, and Valley Fever can cause these virtually anywhere in the body. Valley Fever patients most commonly have lesions in the lung, resulting in diminished lung capacity and coughing up blood in some cases. Naturally, these lesions can also cause more severe problems or even death, because lesions in the lung or any other body part can be dangerous if they grow and progressively destroy organs.

As with cancerous tumors, many cocci lesions need to be surgically removed. In fact, lung cancer is a very common misdiagnosis among many Valley Fever patients with abscesses, cavities, and nodules in their lungs. All of these problems may need resection (the process of cutting away part of the lung) or even lung removal in patients, but this is not always the case. Sometimes the growths caused by Valley Fever can go away on their own or with antifungal drug treatment.

When a doctor sees an x-ray of lung lesions he usually suspects cancer. Testing for Valley Fever is rarely considered. This frequently results in treatment by lung surgery, which is performed much more often than is necessary with Valley Fever.

Many of our questionnaire respondents told us how devastated they and their families were to hear the lung cancer diagnosis, how difficult it was to recover from the lung surgery, and that the doctors later evaluated the tissue removed during surgery and said it was not cancer, but Valley Fever. We have read a lot of frustration over surgeries that may have been totally unnecessary.

We recommend that Valley Fever patients with lung lesions keep copies of their lung x-rays in case a doctor in the future suspects cancer in a lesion known to be caused by Valley Fever. This proactive measure cannot help the people misdiagnosed with lung cancer who unnecessarily lose parts of their lung before they had even heard of this disease, but those who know they are survivors of Valley Fever may be saved from needless surgery, pain, and medical expenses.

People with Valley Fever arthritis often require surgical synovectomy, meaning that the coating around the joint that allows smooth joint movement is removed.

Joint fusion is another medical option for people with bone and joint pain. This medical procedure forces the patient to lose all mobility in the joint in the hope of stopping Valley Fever's destructive action there. If that is not sufficient, amputation of a limb may become necessary. This occurs most often when Valley Fever produces osteomyelitic lesions that destroy the patient's bones.[260]   Very often, doctors use surgery and drugs together.[122]

Drug Basics

While there isn't enough room in this book for all the information on the drugs that are used for Valley Fever treatment, most of the people who contacted us had experienced their side effects.

Surgical side effects are expected because people know a part of their body will be removed along with the fungus and they expect pain or limited mobility as a consequence. The drugs that treat Valley Fever should be treated with equal care. The drugs' side effects increase in severity as their doses increase, and they have side effects that can be "dose limiting." This means that, even if doctors want to use a very high dose of antifungal drugs to fight a severe Valley Fever infection, they may have to limit the drugs to smaller doses because the side effects could become more harmful than the disease itself.[228]   There are frequent medical complaints about the drugs' toxicity.[111]   Other complaints are that the drugs are not effective enough and that they frequently need to be taken for a lifetime.[48]

There are essentially two antifungal drug types used in mainstream coccidioidomycosis therapy.   Amphotericin B formulations are drugs that are normally delivered directly to the veins or cerebrospinal fluid. Azole drugs are typically taken as tablets (pills).

The drugs that treat Valley Fever are all fungistatic, meaning that they can harm the fungus but are not able to kill it completely. They also have a host of side effects, including harm to the liver and kidneys. Dry skin and hair loss are primarily cosmetic side effects, but still unpleasant. Other side effects can lead to major health problems. Spinal taps are done to test the spinal fluid for the possibility of meningitis or to administer intrathecal drugs, but can cause arachnoiditis, a permanent state of ongoing pain from the spine.

A Summary of Drugs Currently Used for Valley Fever

- Amphotericin B — delivered directly to the veins or cerebrospinal fluid
- Azole drugs — typically taken as pills by mouth. Types of Azole Drugs follow:
- Fluconazole (sold as Diflucan)
- Itraconazole (sold as Sporanox)
- Ketoconazole (sold as Nizoral)
- Voriconazole (sold as Vfend)
- Posaconazole (sold as Noxafil). In September 2006 the FDA approved the use of this drug and it seems very promising

Amphotericin B

This drug was developed in the 1950's and came into mainstream use in the 1960's, but amphotericin B remains in use even today. By being inserted intravenously into the patient's bloodstream, it can spread to attack the fungus nearly anywhere. However the blood-brain barrier is not easily crossed, so the drug can also be given as an intrathecal injection. This means it is injected into the spinal fluid that flows between the lining of the brain and spinal cord. By putting the amphotericin B directly into the cerebrospinal fluid it can combat meningitis much more effectively. There is a downside to this treatment, of course.

> "Intrathecal treatments are technically difficult, often produce chemical irritation and discomfort, risk neurologic catastrophe, may engender superinfections of reservoirs or other implanted apparatus, and are not always effective. Clearly, safer and more effective therapies are needed."[101]

Amphotericin B earned the nickname "Ampho-terrible" early in its deployment and that term has even survived to this day due to its horrible side effects. Side effects can increase in severity as the dose of the drug is increased and can include "pain at the site of injection, fevers, chills, nausea, vomiting, electrolyte abnormalities, and nephrotoxicity [kidney damage]."[25]

Other well known side effects include diarrhea, pains in the back, legs or other places, tingling sensations, blurred vision, seizures, fatigue, loss of appetite, shortness of breath, skin rashes, itching, difficult urination, irregular heartbeat, unnatural bleeding or bruising. These do not even complete the list of side effects. "Other side effects not listed above may also occur in some patients. If you notice any other effects, check with your doctor."[176]

The side effects can be treated with other drugs. Antihistamines and acetaminophen were specifically mentioned, along with the highly risky use of corticosteroids.[112]

A typical treatment period with amphotericin B lasts six months[79] but it may be required for a lifetime in other patients.[140] This means there is plenty of time for a patient to experience the horrific side effects. Unfortunately, the treatment can have "substantial neurotoxic effects such as arachnoiditis that may limit treatment and mimic active infection."[113]

Since arachnoiditis is an inflammation of parts of the membrane around the spinal cord and brain, it can be likened very much to meningitis. It is caused by punctures of the spine in spinal taps and intrathecal treatment, rather than by the chemicals in the drug itself. An arachnoiditis support web page stated the problem simply enough: "The biggest complaint of those that suffer from [arachnoiditis] is pain. Unbearable, chronic pain. 24 hours a day. 7 days a week. 52 weeks a year. It is a bleak picture, but those are the facts."[125]

Other neurological problems seen as "common" side effects in patients treated with amphotericin B are:

- Foot drop (a weakness or paralysis of foot muscles. When a person with foot drop tries to walk, toes tend to drag on the ground)
- Paraparesis (a partial paralysis of the legs)
- Double vision
- Hearing loss
- Partial paralysis of facial nerves (nerve paresis)
- Facial pain
- Seizures
- Degenerative brain disease (known as toxic encephalopathy)

"These side effects are most often transient, the usual duration being less than 24 hours. Although occasionally more severe neurological complications may last up to 2 weeks, they are rarely permanent."[140]

While many tests show these side effects in the classic amphotericin B formulation known as Fungizone, there are also many newer formulations that seem to be better tolerated by patients.[25, 243]

Often these are lipid based in their formula, rather than Fungizone's detergent mixture. Lipids are oily, fatty compounds that are essential parts of living cells like proteins and carbohydrates. Their inclusion in amphotericin B formulas seem to reduce side effects and improve treatment tolerance. A wide variety of amphotericin B formulations are available, some of which may be more effective or have fewer side effects than others or the classic "Fungizone" amphotericin B formulation.[2, 25, 51, 93, 154, 243]

If you know someone who is being given amphotericin B, it might be worthwhile to ask the doctor whether it is a lipid formulation. If not, ask if the use of a lipid formulation or another drug might be more effective or have less severe side effects.

Amphotericin B dosages for Valley Fever patients have been written as "0.5 mg/kg." This is a medical shorthand for saying that amphotericin B would be given at half a milligram of the drug per kilogram of the patient's mass for each dose. For the metric conversion, one pound of weight is about 0.45 kilograms of mass. For example, a 150-pound person is equivalent to 68 kilograms, and would receive 0.5 milligrams (mg) of amphotericin B per kilogram of body mass. The dosage would be 34 mg in this example.

A typical dose of amphotericin B with its classic deoxycholate "Fungizone" formulation would be between 0.5 mg/kg and 1.5 mg/kg intravenously each day or on alternate days. The newer lipid formulations could have higher dosages between 2 mg/kg and 5 mg/kg or more.

Side effects are extremely important considerations when placing amphotericin B into the cerebrospinal fluid intrathecally. "The intrathecal dosage of amphotericin B normally ranges between 0.1 mg and 1.5 mg per dose, administered at intervals ranging from daily to weekly, beginning at a low dosage and increasing the size of the dosage until the appearance of patient intolerance (indicated by severe vomiting, prostration, or transient dose-related mental status)."[98]

In intravenous and intrathecal amphotericin B treatments, the time between doses is often increased as symptoms subside. For example, three treatments a week could be lessened to two and then one treatment per week. We have been in contact with Valley Fever patients who must receive amphotericin B treatments for the rest of their lives.

With the pain of the drug and the inconvenience and expense of hospital treatments, azole drugs may be the next step for a patient on amphotericin B. If a patient can be taken off amphotericin B, both the doctor and patient are often glad to switch to azole therapy.

Azole Drugs

Most Valley Fever prescriptions are for azole drugs. The most commonly used azole drugs for this disease are fluconazole (marketed as Diflucan), itraconazole (Sporanox), ketoconazole (Nizoral) and more recently voriconazole (Vfend). The azole drug posaconazole (Noxafil) was recently approved for use and seems very promising.[182]

Azoles can be taken as pills at home so they do not require a hospital setting as amphotericin B often does. Some have been shown to be more effective against some cases of meningitis than amphotericin B and may show a lower likelihood of side effects.

Unfortunately, azole drugs also share many side effects with amphotericin B and have a slew of their own. Liver destruction, kidney destruction, fatal drug interactions, vision problems, hair loss and a host of other problems form a mosaic of horrible side effects that rivals cocci itself.

Side effects that are common among the azole drugs are nausea, vomiting, dizziness, fatigue, abdominal pains, and headaches. The liver damage frequently caused by azole drugs can be recognized by the patient if odd colored stool, dark colored urine, or a yellowish tint to the eyes or skin are noticed.

The allergic reactions to these drugs can manifest as rashes, hives, and swelling of the throat, lips, or tongue.[256] Depending upon the medical source, these symptoms may be considered the drugs' "side effects" instead of an allergic response.[176] Azole drugs can cause birth defects and harm developing babies. This means they cannot be taken by pregnant women. Women who are nursing also cannot use azoles because the drug would be passed through the breast milk to the baby.[256]

Even worse, some azole studies show "relapse rates as high as 75% after only 1 year of stopping therapy."[48] For many with Valley Fever, lifelong azole therapy is considered necessary to avoid relapse.[99]

Doses for most azole drugs are typically written as 400 mg/d, meaning 400 milligrams each day, sometimes split as two 200 mg doses during the day.[98]

Besides the side effects, financial hardships can be a problem. Drug costs are estimated to be $5,000-$20,000 for each year of medication.[99]

For someone who lives over 50 years with lifetime antifungal treatment at this price and doesn't even include additional costs like hospitalization and various appointments with physicians, that person's medication costs would still surpass **one million dollars**. With additional expenses, the financial burden would only get worse.

Ketoconazole

While shared side effects are common among azole drugs, some have specific and noteworthy reactions. Men who might take ketoconazole should know it can cause an inhibition of natural testosterone and potentially can lead to gynecomastia. Gynecomastia is the abnormal and potentially painful enlargement of male breasts.[203]

Ketoconazole can also cause:

- Gastric distress
- Scalp hair loss
- Leukopenia (abnormally decreased presence of white blood cells, which is very serious when fighting Valley Fever)
- Thrombocytosis (increased platelets in the blood)

It can occasionally even cause the onset of osteomyelitis (painful bone inflammation) from the drug, and this type of osteomyelitis was not thought to be the type caused by Valley Fever itself.[37]

While ketoconazole still seems to be given to animals with Valley Fever, our questionnaire responses indicate that in recent years it is almost never prescribed for human patients with this disease.

Itraconazole

Itraconazole appeared to be slightly more effective than fluconazole at fighting skeletal cocci infections, but its use "must be weighed against potential difficulties with absorption and drug interactions, which may limit the usefulness of itraconazole for some patients."[102]

Itraconazole's other side effects include difficulty concentrating, hypokalemia (abnormally low blood potassium which can be lethal in severe cases),[102] nerve palsies (tremors and paralysis),[48] nerve pains, and congestive heart failure symptoms that may include shortness of breath or chest pains.[256]

In 2001, an FDA Public Health Advisory warned that itraconazole could cause congestive heart failure and reaffirmed the potential for liver damage after a series of deaths.[85] These deadly side effects have caught the attention of lawyers who have web sites dedicated to evaluating and suing over the damages caused by itraconazole.

There are apparently dozens of web sites that support litigation based on the side effects of itraconazole. As with the links following our gadolinium information, we are not associated with these sites in any way and are only listing them to demonstrate the kinds of legal assistance available. Many other legal sites seeking clients for severe itraconazole side effect law suits can be found by using an Internet search engine.

http://www.rwklaw.com/lamisil_sporanox.shtml
http://www.apinjurylaw.com/lamisil_sporanox.shtml
http://www.jpgslaw.com/stores/741/sporanox.cfm
http://www.legalmatch.com/law-library/article/sporanox-lawyers.html

Fluconazole

Fluconazole is sold under the name Diflucan and was established for use against cocci in the 1990's. Fluconazole's side effects include hair loss (notably more so than with itraconazole), anorexia, tinnitus (buzzing or ringing in the ears), dry skin, and unnatural drowsiness. It is thought that fluconazole might be more effective than previous azoles against meningitis as doses are increased because it is absorbed well, but doctors noted "the possibility exists that as yet unforeseen chronic neurologic complications of persistent low-level infection may arise."[101]

Fluconazole was the most commonly prescribed drug in Valley Fever Survivor questionnaires. It has replaced amphotericin B in many meningitis cases since the 1990's and was considered "preferred" to the other antifungal drugs in Valley Fever treatment guidelines, particularly when the patient's symptoms are not rapidly worsening.[99] Other doctors disagree and prefer amphotericin B for meningitis cases,[63] but Valley Fever cases are often so different from one another that it may be difficult to decide.

Azoles Vs. Amphotericin B

As noted above, there are differing opinions about which drug may be best for Valley Fever treatment. Azole drugs have been used to treat cocci meningitis, but amphotericin B may be more effective in some cases.[29,79] Azole drugs, particularly fluconazole, have been recommended for treatment of meningitis caused by Valley Fever[99] but the drug selection may vary on a case-to-case basis. Other doctors still refer to amphotericin B as the "gold standard"[80] and "the drug of choice for the treatment of coccidioidomycosis,"[109] especially when meningitis is involved. Unfortunately, amphotericin B is only considered to successfully help symptoms of "coccidioidal meningitis in <25% of cases."[113]

A New Generation of Antifungal Drugs

While the drugs above are well known in the world of Valley Fever, new antifungal drugs have been developed. These were originally used against other fungal diseases first and later tested for effectiveness against *Coccidioides*.

Even with the limited testing that has already occurred, prescribing them for patients with this disease is considered an "off label" drug use due to the lack of in-depth study. None of the following three drugs have gone through the stringent evaluation necessary to determine their overall safety in Valley Fever infections. Also, after various drug safety scandals, it is possible that the prescription of drugs for "off label" use may be limited in the future.

Posaconazole

Posaconazole (marketed as Noxafil) may have less toxic effects on the liver than other azole drugs. Posaconazole has even been shown to be as effective as itraconazole at one tenth the dose.[109] It is also known to penetrate the blood-brain barrier, making it useful for meningitis cases.[201]

> "Posaconazole was 50- to 200-fold more potent than fluconazole and itraconazole at preventing death and reducing fungal burden" in experiments with mice, and may also be a more effective alternative to these drugs in human cases.[182]

Many of the azole drugs share unpleasant side effects. While posaconazole has many of these, it also may cause lowered white blood cell counts,[84] which can be a problem for Valley

Fever recovery. Posaconazole was only authorized for use in other fungal diseases by the FDA in 2006 so additional side effects may also be discovered as Valley Fever patients take it. However, its effectiveness and reduced burden on the liver show promise that it may become a mainstay of Valley Fever treatment.

Voriconazole

Voriconazole (marketed as Vfend) is another of the newer drugs. It may also be more powerful than fluconazole against Valley Fever, but with side effects that involve sensitivity to light, blurry vision, or virtual loss of vision that may require that its users stop driving or operating machinery.[58] One questionnaire respondent temporarily experienced complete blindness while on voriconazole, but her vision recovered when she stopped taking the drug.

Some patients taking voriconazole had suffered squamous cell carcinoma on their skin. This is a type of malignant tumor that followed the severe sensitivity to sunlight that developed in some patients taking the drug. In one case where a woman suffered from this after three years on voriconazole, and after the "radical destructive surgery" on her face to remove the tumors, she was switched to posaconazole treatment. Her photosensitivity reaction completely went away.[173]

Due to the risk of carcinoma in patients who have the photosensitivity reaction, "an alternate [antifungal] agent should be used whenever possible."[173]

Since Valley Fever poses so much of a problem for people with compromised immune systems, it is also worth noting that voriconazole should not be used with the HIV drugs ritonavir and efavirenz, as this can produce undesirable drug interactions. "While posaconazole is probably safe, more information is needed before it can be recommended" but "fluconazole and itraconazole are probably safe to use" for patients who must also use these HIV medications.[5]

Both posaconazole and voriconazole are increasingly being given to Valley Fever patients. These drugs have been considered "hundreds of times more potent than ketoconazole as antifungals"[55] and have been effective even in cases where high doses of fluconazole or even amphotericin B did not appear to help the patient.[182]

Caspofungin

Caspofungin (marketed as Cancidas) is an intravenous antifungal drug that is not from the azole group. Its primary method of action is to destroy the beta glucan in the cell walls of fungi.[108, 126] While caspofungin has shown effectiveness against Valley Fever in experimental mice and in vitro studies,[108] and it may be helpful in combination with other drugs against Valley Fever,[196] effectiveness on its own may be dubious in human patients.

One experimental case involved a 23-year-old African American truck driver who was believed to have been infected while driving through Arizona. He suffered through meningitis and other Valley Fever symptoms with ineffective high dose treatments of fluconazole and voriconazole. When amphotericin B treatment was tried but was found to be too toxic for his kidneys, he was placed on caspofungin to see if it would help. It was tried for 22 days but the drug failed to help. The young man died shortly after treatment was restarted with other drugs.

> "...our experience would make us reluctant to use caspofungin at the current standard dose in patients with coccidioidomycosis."[126]

This patient obviously had a severe case and was in a high risk group, so this is not to say the drug is completely ineffective, only unproven in the treatment of Valley Fever.

We could not locate a record of further attempts with caspofungin alone treating other Valley Fever cases. While the drug is known to help patients with other fungi, it still needs to be considered experimental for this disease.

The Vaccine and Cure Projects

Other important drugs that are further on the horizon and not presently ready for commercial use may be the most important.

The Valley Fever Vaccine Project

The Valley Fever Vaccine Project (VFVP) is an academic-based consortium of public and private interests dedicated to developing a vaccine to prevent the disease.

- California State University, Bakersfield, Foundation serves as a primary contractor and holds the commercialization rights to the vaccine.
- University of California Office of the President serves as the licensing agent for the vaccine.
- University of California/San Francisco provides day-to-day project management and oversight of the intellectual property portfolio of the VFVP.
- Research and development team comprised of scientists from University of Arizona, University of Kansas, University of Texas/San Antonio, University of California/Davis, University of California/San Diego, and Medical University of Ohio.

The VFVP has received funds from the Centers for Disease Control and Prevention, State of California Department of Health Services, California HealthCare Foundation, County of Kern, Valley Fever Americas Foundation (VFAF) and other regional non-profit organizations. Hundreds of private individuals have contributed to the VFAF in amounts ranging from $5 to $15,000. The VFAF is a broad community-based effort supporting the vaccine effort developed by Rotarians in District 5240, which includes the Rotary Clubs in District 5240 of Rotary International (which include Bakersfield and other heavily endemic areas in California).

Several different vaccine candidates have been developed by scientists funded by the VFVP. At the time of this writing, the VFAF is focusing on a fusion protein vaccine that combines two antigens (rAg2/PRA1-106 and rCsa). If successful, this vaccine will sensitize the immune system to Valley Fever so a vaccinated person can mount an immune defense if any *Coccidioides* spores are inhaled.

Early testing with this vaccine shows a 97% survival rate in mice given an otherwise lethal dose. Although the fusion protein vaccine also offered some protection in primate trials, it "did not prevent pulmonary disease."[118] There are also manufacturing difficulties that must be overcome before this vaccine candidate can succeed.

The UTSA Vaccine Research

A vaccine project headed by Dr. Garry Cole at the University of Texas at San Antonio (UTSA) may not only work to stop people from contracting Valley Fever but may even be able to benefit or cure those who are already infected.

In Dr. Cole's project, he developed vaccines that are actually "live attenuated mutant strains" of *Coccidioides*, genetically designed so that they cannot produce chitin, the material that makes fungal cell walls. This Δchs5 strain can grow as mycelia but not as a parasitic spherule or endospore, crippling its ability to act as a parasite.[54]   In vaccines such as Δchs5, the triangle would be read as the Greek letter "delta" and each letter and number would be pronounced.

A different genetically engineered vaccine candidate known as the "triple mutant" Δcts2/Δard1/Δcts3 strain can become a spherule but does not produce endospores. In either case, without the ability to reproduce, these fungi are neutralized. The body can recognize them, however, and can then mount an immune response against natural *Coccidioides*.

In a test, 80 dangerous arthroconidial spores were given intranasally to a group of mice that had been vaccinated with the attenuated triple mutant strain and a group that had not been vaccinated. 100% of the vaccinated mice survived up to the end of the study at 75 days, while 100% of the non-vaccinated mice died within 16 days.[118]

Some might wonder whether this live fungal vaccine is safe. In a demonstration with the triple mutant strain, mice were experimentally infected with doses up to 5,000 spores. None showed evidence of sickness.[118]

The attenuated mutant spores may serve as a vaccine and are considered safe. In fact, the CDC does not consider the spores hazardous enough to keep the triple mutant strain on the List of Select Agents and Toxins, as it does with the naturally occurring *C. immitis* and *C. posadasii* strains.[39]

Nikkomycin Z

The FDA has approved one million dollars for study of the drug nikkomycin Z, which may be a cure. It is currently being evaluated at the University of Arizona.

Nikkomycin Z is a drug created in the 1970's and was shown in the 1980's and 1990's to be able to inhibit the production of chitin, the material in *Coccidioides* cell walls.[119] Later studies have shown experimental animals' lungs were sterilized (free) of the fungus, meaning nikkomycin Z could be a cure for Valley Fever. In 2005 nikkomycin Z was experimentally shown again to work against *Coccidioides* both alone and with other antifungal drugs.[117]

The drug appears to be promising, but it is worth noting that previous vaccine candidates had been effective in mice but not in humans so there is no guarantee of nikkomycin Z's effectiveness. In 2005 the University of Arizona finally acquired rights to nikkomycin Z with the intent to research its effectiveness, but as much as $100 million may be required to test this proposed cure and bring it to market.

Roadblocks

Vaccine research has faced stop-and-go funding over the years, and rights to the drug nikkomycin Z have been shuffled from one organization to another over the course of decades.

If nikkomycin Z worked flawlessly as a cure, were fully funded, and were fast tracked for approval, 5-7 years would be the soonest it could appear on the general market.[96] Under the best case assumption that all goes well for the current vaccine research projects, a similar time frame could be expected. More details on these experimental projects will be included in our upcoming book.

We hope that the vaccine and cure projects will truly be effective and advocate that these worthwhile endeavors can be financed completely. Please read Appendix A: Organizations and Internet Resources to learn how you can help these organizations with their research.

Drug Interactions

Drug interactions are another major concern. Most of the antifungal drugs are generally known to cause side effects on the patient's liver, and also may have adverse effects with other drugs. For example, Dr. Craig Rundbaken (who treated roughly 300 Valley Fever patients in Sun City West, Arizona in 2007) told us that patients taking Coumadin (warfarin) before their Valley Fever diagnosis had to reduce their doses by 75% when fluconazole was prescribed.

Although some antibacterial antibiotics can cause devastating effects in patients with cocci on their own, they can also combine with antifungal drugs to lessen the patient's immune response[132] which could become a devastating or lethal development.[48]

If you must take an antifungal drug like the ones mentioned in this chapter, it is urgent that you don't simply read a printed page in a book to see which drugs should not be taken with them, but rather to get the most updated information possible. Privately owned web sites like the following may be helpful. These are only a handful of the sites available with this information, and any web search for drug information will probably yield many more sources of information.

http://www.druginfonet.com
http://www.familydoctor.org
http://www.mayohealth.org
http://www.medicinenet.com
http://www.netwellness.org
http://www.rxlist.com
http://www.webmd.com

The following U.S. Government web sites also provide searchable drug information that can be helpful for keeping up to date.

http://chid.nih.gov
http://www.healthfinder.gov
http://www.fda.gov/cder/consumerinfo/default.htm
http://medlineplus.gov/
http://www.nlm.nih.gov/medlineplus/druginformation.html

We encourage you to use this information as a starting point, to visit several sites, and always consult with your doctor about what you find.

While caring doctors may be impressed to see their patients educating themselves, others may not be. If your doctor is offended at the fact that you are taking a proactive role in your health care, don't let it bother you. Your health matters more than your doctor's ego. Your doctor may even appreciate learning something new about these drugs and their side effects.

Dosage Issues

Higher doses of a drug are expected to make the side effects worse. A fairly standard dose of azole drug therapy is 400 mg per day. When cases do not improve on this dose, especially when patients have meningitis symptoms that resist lower dose treatment, 800 mg per day have been tried, as well as even higher doses from 1200-2000 mg per day.

Sometimes even these high doses do not help fight the disease but instead produce unwanted side effects in the nervous system and other organs,[58] especially the liver, that potentially make these high doses of the drugs lethal.

If a patient has severe meningitis that isn't responding to amphotericin B or azole therapy, perhaps high doses or combinations of the drugs may be able to help. However, it has occasionally been reported by our Valley Fever questionnaire respondents that their doctors wanted to write a report about the experimental effectiveness of high dose antifungal drugs. It is a style of medical treatment that may be viewed as putting the patient into the circumstances of a guinea pig rather than as a person to be healed.

Regardless of the circumstances of your need for Valley Fever treatment, ask if any of your physicians will be writing about your case in a medical journal or speaking about it at a conference. Although it is good to add to the body of scientific knowledge and peer reviewed medical journals do not use patients' names in case reports, you can ask them not write about your case if you prefer.

If you are being given unusually high doses of antifungal drugs, you should agree with your doctor that this treatment is necessary. For example, your case could be so severe that you need these high doses, and then you could consider the increased likelihood of the drugs' side effects as a calculated risk. You always have the right to refuse to take experimental drugs or dosages, and to ask your doctor if there are other treatment options.

Be sure that you ask questions about your treatment to find out whether there is anything unorthodox, unusual, or experimental about your treatment. You should be comfortable with the care you receive. If you are uncomfortable with any treatment plan set out for you, you have the right to seek a second opinion.

Easing the Expense

With the high cost of antifungal drugs, whether you are a human patient or trying to help an animal receive medication, there are significant ways you may be able to reduce your costs. Some of these have been brought to us as tips from Valley Fever survivors who wanted to share their minor victories over the costs of medicine.

Samples

Doctors and veterinarians are often given small promotional packages of drugs to give out as "samples" to their patients when they feel it appropriate. It may be worthwhile to ask whether your doctor has samples of the VF drug you are prescribed, or if he can get some for you. Aside from the fact that each dose is free, there may be a major cost savings if the doctor wants to switch you to another drug. The expense of a full prescription would not have been wasted if the medication was ineffective for your infection or if your body could not tolerate its side effects.

Valuable Insurance Information

Erica S. shared some of the following advice about a policy that may benefit many who have switched their insurance companies.

An FYI for anyone who has had to switch insurance companies for one reason or another during a calendar year: Anything paid towards your deductible for Company A can be applied towards your deductible for Company B.

For example, my deductible with Company A was $350, my new one is $500. Not knowing this, I've paid more than $500 already thinking I had to meet a new deductible. So now $350 will be applied to out of pocket expenses with my new company. This is in the state of Arizona, I don't know about other states but my sister-in-law in Ohio told me about it, so it may be true elsewhere too.

The numerous phone calls and faxes and letters required for this can be overwhelming. Perhaps an attorney to sort out this mess would have been better! My husband has been making all the calls, so I am very thankful for that.

You need to request a Continuance of Coverage with the NEW insurance company. They should approve you for a set number of appointments with the same doctor you were seeing under your old insurance company, at their in-network level (my husband was told this is a federal law, the number of visits may vary between states). Once those visits run out (for example, they gave us 8 visits from 12/1 - 1/31), you can request additional visits, but you may have to prove why your doctors are more capable at treating you than their in-network doctors. We included the print out from Mayo's website re: their Cocci Clinic, and that was sufficient.

You also need a copy of the actual policy (NOT the little one page summary they try to pass off as the policy)—if you have this insurance policy from work, check with the human resources department. You may have this already. Good grief we had to pull teeth to get it.

Also, it might help to get the sales rep who sold the policy involved. It's in their best interest to help you, and they may be able to do something quickly as well.

Knowing the expenses for doctor visits, labs, etc for VF can be enormous, hopefully this can help save someone some money.

This opportunity may not be advertised upfront so you should check your own policy to find out whether this applies in your case.

Pharmaceutical Philanthropy

When you ask about samples, you may also wish to ask your doctor whether the pharmaceutical companies would be willing to give you the drugs you need for free. The companies that produce and normally sell their drugs are willing to give their products away free of charge or at a reduced cost to some patients that cannot afford their prescribed medication.

The Partnership for Prescription Assistance (PPA) is a coalition of pharmaceutical companies that understand not everyone can afford the drugs they make. They can help some people who cannot afford their medicine by providing it free or at a low cost. Their web site required browser cookies at the time of my visit or it would not display anything but a blank white screen. With cookies enabled, there was information about this service here:

http://www.pparx.org

The Partnership for Prescription Assistance can also be reached through their telephone number 1-888-4PPA-NOW (1-888-477-2669).

Other programs like the Pfizer Patient Assistance Programs listed below may help, and other companies' plans may also be available.

http://www.pfizer.com/pfizer/subsites/philanthropy/access/us.programs.index.jsp

https://www.pfizerhelpfulanswers.com/ProgramList.aspx

Many of these programs can only be enacted at a doctor's request so you must ask your doctor if there is any plan available for the type of medication you need and if he or she will be willing to make this request for you. If you are not able to succeed with one plan, ask your doctors to suggest other plans you may be eligible for, as they might be aware of other groups that might help reduce prescription costs.

Veterinary Assistance

If your pet has a severe case of Valley Fever and you simply can't afford medical treatment, ask your veterinarian about free samples of the drugs prescribed. Also contact your local animal control organizations and even nearby veterinary schools for help. If they cannot provide you with the medication your pet needs, ask if they know of anyone who might.

In addition, www.imom.org may be an invaluable website. IMOM is an organization dedicated to helping animals that would otherwise die due to lack of funds for their veterinary expenses or medication.

Tips for Buying Medicine

While comparison shopping is always useful, we have been informed that purchases at hospital pharmacies have been dramatically more expensive than the same drug purchases at ordinary pharmacies. Further, we have been told that warehouse club stores (Costco, Sam's Club, etc.) often have pharmacies with prescription drugs sold at lower prices than patients can find elsewhere.

Call your local club stores to check their prices. If you are not a member or not able to become a member, call or visit your local warehouse club store and ask if the pharmacy can be used by non-members. Often it can.

Regardless of eligibility for any drug program, also be sure to ask your doctor for recommendations about ways to get the medication at an affordable price.

Since lower cost generic versions of some Valley Fever drugs are available, you may wish to speak with your doctor about taking a generic form of the drug.

Beyond Medical Care

At a Glance

- People may help to fight Valley Fever by reducing stress and improving their diet.
- Physical therapy may play a role in Valley Fever recovery.
- Some non-medical remedies may be dangerous.

Stress and the Immune System

People with Valley Fever often ask what they can do to help their bodies fight the disease or to improve their lives. Aside from proper medical care, it seems important that people work to make their general health as good as it can be. This way, even when Valley Fever causes further problems, the effect on people's overall health and quality of life can be minimized as much as possible.

The immune response plays a major role in fighting off Valley Fever, so immunity is an important area of focus. Some medications like steroids can suppress the immune system. Stress reduction may be important to Valley Fever patients because mental stress is known to adversely affect the immune system.[1, 161] Naturally, some Valley Fever patients may find it difficult to relax when they discover they've been infected with an incurable fungal parasite that can reactivate at any time.

Fortunately, there are some simple health promoting and immune system boosting actions that anyone can take.

The Alkaline Diet Concept

Diet plays a strong role in our health, but to date we are unaware of any medical research studies into diet and Valley Fever. With that said, once Sharon began to "come back to the world of the living" from her severe case of Valley Fever, she realized the need to do whatever it takes to bolster her health in order to keep fighting this disease.

Sharon believed that an alkaline diet would be beneficial and started to research the subject. Since that time we have found that several nutritionists have suggested an "alkaline diet" strategy for good health in general, although not specifically in relation to Valley Fever. People on an alkaline diet eat more foods that are said to be metabolized by the body to create a more chemically alkaline environment in the bloodstream, and less of the foods that are said to create an acid environment. Theoretically, this reduces the levels of harmful acid in the body.

The foods said to produce an alkalizing effect are most vegetables, nuts, berries, and soy. Foods that lead to a more acidifying effect are meats, egg yolks, most grains, breads, cheeses, sugary foods, junk foods, etc. Many complete food lists can be found on the web when searching for the term "alkaline diet" or for words like "alkaline foods" and "acid foods" (although some lists contradict one another on some items). The general concept of the alkaline diet has been promoted by a variety of people, from motivational speaker Anthony Robbins, naturopath Robert Young, and even the "Sleeping Psychic" Edgar Cayce.

This dietary theory is not entirely without caveats. Blood alkalinity is not known to change significantly based on dietary intake; rather it is stable like one's body temperature. There is even disagreement as to whether certain foods on the lists are actually "alkaline" in the process of metabolism. For example, oranges have a high citric acid content but are said to promote alkalinity in virtually every variation of this diet.

Most importantly, even if this diet truly could create a more alkaline pH in the body, that change would not necessarily be desirable for Valley Fever patients. When parasitic *Coccidioides* spherules are reproducing as endospores, they release an alkalizing compound that helps keep them safer from the body's immune defenses.[127, 183]

Regardless of any controversies with the diet's theory of alkalization, this type of diet has a greater focus on vegetables and nutrient rich foods than the standard American diet. Since many of these foods have been scientifically proven to be rich in antioxidants and to provide anti-inflammatory benefits (explained later in this chapter), while most of the "acid" foods are not known to produce these benefits, the dietary concept should be considered.

Although she was completely healthy before her Valley Fever infection, co-author Sharon improved her diet with this method afterward. She finds that this has helped her, and all others with Valley Fever who gave up eating sugary foods and began eating an "alkaline diet," have also reported that they found it to produce a noticeable improvement in their general health.

Probiotics

There is scientific proof of an immune-boosting benefit of probiotic supplements.[3] Literally meaning "promoting life" as opposed to antibiotics ("anti-life"), probiotic supplements and foods contain live cultures of a variety of bacteria that benefit our immune systems.

Yogurt made from cultured milk is the most famous probiotic food, although products similar to dairy yogurt may also be made of cultured soy and other ingredients. Kefir is a thick, carbonated, cultured dairy beverage that is also probiotic. It can often be found in health food stores.

Before purchasing a probiotic food, be sure that the label specifically says it has live and active cultures within the product. If it were simply *made* with live and active cultures, it might not contain them later due to ingredients or processes that add flavor or lengthen its shelf life. Plain yogurt and kefir products are healthier than those with added sugars.

Probiotic supplement pills are likely to assist the process even better than probiotic foods if they are able to provide more "active cultures" or "Colony Forming Units" (CFU) of beneficial bacteria that arrives at their proper destination during the digestive process. If a probiotic supplement pill does not have an indication of how many billions of CFU it has per dose, it should not be expected to be more beneficial than a probiotic food. Since there is no labeling standardization, CFU could also be called probiotic organisms, cultures, or any other description of these beneficial organisms. "10 billion cultures are included" is intended to mean the same as "a dose of 10 billion CFU," presuming the companies involved measured their products accurately.

The following products are mentioned to help you get started looking for the probiotic supplement that is right for you. We are not associated with any of the companies mentioned. All the information below is based on material supplied by the probiotic supplement manufacturers at their web sites or on their packaging, and many other companies with probiotic products may be available. Consider this information as a starting point for investigation:

Country Life Vitamins produces "Daily Dophilus" probiotic capsule supplements that provide 5.9 billion active cultures in AM and PM pills. www.country-life.com

Dannon's "Danactive" probiotic is a refrigerated beverage with 10 billion active *Lactobacillus casei* cultures. Although most flavors have added sugar, the label claims a very high dose of beneficial bacteria and it may be the most common probiotic supplement for immune health in supermarkets. www.danactive.com

Uni Key Health Systems' "Probiotics 12" capsules provide 1.3 billion cultures per pill and recommend two pills per dose. Their "Flora-Key" product has 6.5 billion cultures per teaspoon of probiotic powder that can be taken with liquids. www.unikeyhealth.com

Vitamin Research Products sells "BioPRO Powder" with 6.5 CFU of probiotic powder in each quarter-tablespoon scoop. Their "BioPRO Capsules" have 1 billion CFU per capsule, and "Culturelle 30" provides 30 billion cultures per capsule. www.vrp.com

Mushrooms for the Immune System

Many studies have shown that specific mushrooms may help to boost the effectiveness of the immune system. Unfortunately, there are no peer reviewed studies that prescribe an exact amount of a particular mushroom, mushroom by-product, or supplement that will cause the desired immunological benefit in a person suffering with Valley Fever or other specific diseases. Not every type of mushroom is safe to eat and not every mushroom is known to boost the immune system's functions, but research studies have demonstrated that shiitake,[267] lingzhi,[268] maitake,[265] and reishi[164] mushrooms have immune-boosting effects. These mushrooms may be a valuable addition to a healthy diet or supplementation plan for a stronger immune system.

Inflammation

Another scientifically researched way for Valley Fever patients (and those with any other disease that causes inflammation) to help themselves naturally is with an anti-inflammatory diet. Valley Fever causes inflammation in many of its disease processes. The body certainly doesn't need more inflammation to deal with.

The foods that people avoid may be just as important as the ones they eat. Although data was not included which would show that a specific amount of sugar would trigger a specific amount of cellular inflammation, refined sugars and other quickly digested carbohydrates like many pastas and flour-based baked goods have been demonstrated to increase inflammatory processes within the body. Saturated fats from animal and dairy products and fried foods also contribute to this process.

This does not mean healthy meals are difficult to make. Green vegetables, berries, fruits, oats, yogurt, kefir, fish, beans and a surprisingly large list of foods can actually decrease these harmful processes. The beneficial effects from these foods have been heavily researched in scientific journals.

Dermatologist Dr. Nicholas Perricone reviewed and distilled much of this medical research into his bestselling books, *The Perricone Promise*,[198] *The Perricone Weight Loss Diet*,[199] and *Dr. Perricone's 7 Secrets to Beauty, Health, and Longevity*.[197] Dr. Perricone notes that the fight against cellular inflammation had tremendous benefits to improve his patients' skin complexion and their ability to lose body fat. The research also shows how these foods are scientifically proven to improve people's health in other important ways, like increased energy and improved immune system function.

An anti-inflammatory diet may not specifically fight Valley Fever. However, if it can remove even a small amount of inflammation that would otherwise have been present, perhaps in a patient with arthritis symptoms, that may be the difference between inconvenient joint pain from Valley Fever and raging "Desert Rheumatism."

As Dr. Perricone's bibliographies and other searches in the medical literature show, the research on benefits of anti-inflammatory foods is extensive and ever-growing. Green tea, for example, is a part of this program and is cited by many researchers for a wide variety of healing benefits. Some scientists evaluated its anti-inflammatory benefits for neurodegenerative disorders.[169] Others have discovered it may even help with sepsis.[46] Sepsis is a blood infection that can occur due to many organisms including *Coccidioides*. With such important benefits being discovered from anti-inflammatory foods, they may be able to help Valley Fever patients in a variety of beneficial ways.

Antioxidants

Antioxidants are substances that can counter damaging effects in bodily tissue. Some of these protective substances are vitamin A, vitamin C, selenium, vitamin E, lycopene (commonly found in tomatoes and paprika) and many others. They have "potential effects in the prevention of chronic and degenerative diseases such as cancer and cardiovascular disease as well as aging."[264]

Antioxidants can prevent and often undo the damage caused by free radicals. Free radicals are unstable molecules in the body that can cause oxidative damage. When one considers that oxidized iron is rust, it paints a vivid picture of the effects of oxidation in your body. Free radicals are important factors in stress, immune dysfunction, disease, and the signs of aging.[8, 186]

Calorie restriction is a well documented way to extend the lives of laboratory mice. It is thought to work because a decreased food intake means less of a chance for foods to create free radicals that would damage and age the body.[251]

Judging by increases in obesity in nearly every nation in the world, calorie restriction does not seem like a likely trend. Fortunately, there are other ways to decrease the level of oxidative damage we may experience. "The association between high intake of fruit and vegetables and low incidence of certain cancers is well established. Dietary antioxidants present in these foods are thought to decrease free radical attack on DNA and hence to protect against mutations that cause cancer" and other health issues.[76]

In a sampling of peer reviewed medical literature, there have been studies on how the antioxidants in kiwi fruit, for example, prevent DNA damage in human immune system cells.[56]

Another experiment in humans showed that beta-carotene (25 mg/day), vitamin C (100 mg/day), and vitamin E (280 mg/day) supplementation was able to help their immune cells (lymphocytes) resist oxidative DNA damage in nonsmokers and even in people who smoked. The oxidative resistance also carried over to the lab when their blood cells faced an artificial oxidation experiment.[76] Astaxanthin, a very powerful antioxidant and anti-inflammatory compound may also have powerful immune system and anticancer benefits.[47, 133, 246]

Since "cellular oxidative stress is a critical step in burn-mediated injury," an experiment was conducted to increase the level of antioxidants as therapy for severe burn victims. Treatment with vitamin C, glutathione, and other antioxidants improved burn victims' survival rates and reduced the severity of their complications.[124]

Antioxidant supplementation had been shown to minimize muscle damage in athletes after heavy training overloads that would normally cause fatigue and muscular breakdown.[192]

> Valley Fever patients will find it significant that "antioxidant supplementation essentially reverses several age-associated immune deficiencies."[151]

The USDA developed the ORAC scale (Oxygen Radical Absorbance Capacity) scale[250] to measure the benefits of antioxidants in certain foods. The ORAC scale shows which foods have the highest ORAC ratings, and therefore have the most antioxidants. Increased intake of antioxidants may be able to fight off the damage caused by free radicals. The chart below[171] can be summarized with "eat your fibrous fruits and vegetables," but specific examples of high ORAC ratings are shown. Each number represents the relative antioxidant value of 100 grams of the food, which is about three and a half ounces.

Foods with high ORAC ratings			
Fruits		*Vegetables*	
Prunes	5770	Kale	1770
Raisins	2830	Spinach	1260
Blueberries	2400	Brussels sprouts	980
Blackberries	2036	Alfalfa sprouts	930
Strawberries	1540	Broccoli flowers	890
Raspberries	1220	Beets	840
Plums	949	Red bell pepper	710
Oranges	750	Onion	450
Red grapes	739	Corn	400
Cherries	670	Eggplant	390
Kiwi fruit	602		
Grapefruit, pink	483		

While labs continue studying the specific reasons that antioxidants are so beneficial, it is plainly clear that antioxidants can benefit the human body and immune system cells. Since a strong immune system is an important step to putting a Valley Fever infection into remission, a diet rich in antioxidant foods is one more important step that can benefit your health.

The information here on nutrition is not simply something for a grocery list. Medical considerations are being made to apply probiotics, antioxidants, blood sugar regulation, and other nutrition-related factors even in intensive care settings due to the "rapidly expanding landscape of knowledge" of their benefits.[220] Proper nutrition may be an important way to help your body in its fight against Valley Fever.

Physical Therapy

Beyond the drugs, surgeries, and foods that can aid in healing, exercise can play a role in recovery from Valley Fever. Presuming that the symptoms have sufficiently gone into remission that the patient can begin exercising, an exercise program is often recommended and then supervised by a physical therapist specializing in lung or heart care. Aerobic activity is typically used to help fight off the fatigue. When the symptoms of fatigue are not as noticeable and the patient has greater endurance through improvements in blood pressure, heart rate, and other metrics, then other exercises can be gradually introduced.

> "Neurologic damage or bone and joint involvement may require physical or occupational therapy rehabilitation and depends on what nerves are affected by the disease. If coccidioidomycosis results in bone and joint involvement, the rehabilitation program begins once pain and other symptoms subside. This is followed by range-of-motion exercises to return joint mobility."[175]

Since every patient's case of Valley Fever can affect different organs, one should expect that every patient's physical therapy program could be different as well. Further, many of the problems that Valley Fever causes can be in parts of the body that limit the ability to exercise.

Some people who contacted Valley Fever Survivor had another concern about physical therapy: The body heat it generates.

Raising Your Body Temperature

We had been asked this question about physical activity:

> "*Coccidioides* spores grow in hot places like the desert southwest. Will it protect me from a Valley Fever reactivation if I avoid hot beverages and exercises that raise my body temperature?"

No. While San Joaquin Valley Fever is named as much for the primary location of its earliest recorded outbreaks as for the fever it can produce, the human body's temperature is very stable. If someone chooses to drink cold water the body will just burn slightly more calories to maintain an even body temperature. If the drink is hot water instead, the body will burn slightly fewer calories to maintain the same internal temperature. The same is true of the body's reaction for people living in slightly warmer or slightly colder climates.

Some Valley Fever patients have been instructed to exercise as a part of their therapy to overcome some of their symptoms. Other patients, such as those with coccidioidal arthritis, have been told exercise might make their symptoms worse. The internal human body temperature normally remains fairly constant, even during exercise. We have found absolutely no research to indicate exercise could cause a reactivation or increase *Coccidioides* growth in the body. However, if you are ill and overstress your body with too much exercise or uncomfortable temperatures, your case could get worse due to the effects of stress but not the heat.

Of course, unless someone has specific medical reasons not to exercise, most health experts agree that moderate exercise is generally beneficial.

An Unproven and Dangerous Self-Remedy

There are claims on the Internet that sulfur (flowers of sulfur or sublimed sulfur) can cure Valley Fever. Please be aware we could find no medical research on the validity of these claims. This elemental sulfur is unrelated to "sulfa" drugs (sulfonamides), and there can be serious side effects if sulfur is ingested. Warning labels on sulfur packages have stated that it is not for ingestion. No doctor to our knowledge has ever suggested a person take this toxic, explosive substance to treat Valley Fever.

Some people with Valley Fever had tried this "cure" and dismissed their unpleasant reactions to the sulfur. This is because they heard some fungi release toxins when they die, and they assume their new problems will go away once all the *Coccidioides* fungi are dead. This is known as the Herxheimer reaction, but does not apply to Valley Fever because the fungi of *Coccidioides* spp. do not release these toxins and have not been tested for vulnerability to ingested sulfur. Sulfur is therefore the likely cause of the discomfort. We do not have any follow-up information to know if or how seriously the people were hurt by the sulfur.

Further, some people are allergic to sulfur. In our interview with Robert J. Brauer Jr., then the Executive Director of the Valley Fever Center for Excellence, he stated, "Sulfur treatment [for Valley Fever] is basically taking a toxic chemical and putting it into your system, like sulfuric acid." We do not recommend the use of sulfur for this disease.

In one of our web site's animal surveys, we were told of a dog owner who insisted on "natural treatment," meaning the sulfur that had been suggested on the web. He claimed the dog was "cured" with the sulfur treatment, but it died later due to respiratory failure from a lung lesion—the pet owner apparently did not know that lung lesions are common Valley Fever symptoms. Tragically, had the dog been treated with antifungal medication that is known to work instead of the "sulfur cure," its life might have been spared.

Valley Fever in Animals

The wide variety of symptoms noted in the Symptoms Chapter also apply to Valley Fever in animals. Since animals can't express that they have these problems as clearly as humans can, pet owners should watch their animals' behavior for an indication of those symptoms and especially the symptoms below.

What to look for

Animals with Valley Fever can display some, all, or occasionally none of the following symptoms:[139, 238]

- Weight Loss
- Lameness/limping
- Poor appetite
- Coughing
- Bone Pain
- Spinal Pain

- Fatigue
- Vision loss
- Seizures
- Change in Behavior
- Change in Personality
- Not acting well or being inactive

If your pet shows some of these symptoms and lives in or has visited an endemic area, we recommend you contact your veterinarian and suggest the possibility of a coccidioidomycosis infection. This could save your pet's life.

Any animal has an equal opportunity to inhale a *Coccidioides* spp. spore since they have to breathe as well. However, some dog species tend to get severe cases more easily. "Breeds that may be overrepresented include the Boxer, Pointer, Australian Shepherd, Beagle, Scottish Terrier, Doberman Pinscher, and Cocker Spaniel."[155] Whether they are purebred or mixed bred dogs does not matter, they can suffer extremely serious and even fatal cases of Valley Fever.

"In disseminated disease, the bones and joints are the most frequent targets. In these cases, lameness is the most common symptom. Occasionally, the fungus may invade the brain and seizures can result."[225]

Greyhounds also suffer from Valley Fever frequently.[238] They usually show symptoms of bone lesions and weight loss, but all their pet owner may notice is that they just don't feel well. Other dogs tend to have lung and bone disease manifest equally with Valley Fever.

If you own a Whippet or Greyhound with Valley Fever, he or she may need to be force-fed while on antifungal medication. These breeds tend to lose their appetite and cannot afford to lose any more weight. If they do, they may perish. Dr. Suzanne Stack is a veterinarian who provided specific force-feeding directions here:
https://home.comcast.net/~greyhndz/tips.htm

Medical care

If your dog shows any signs of this disease, please take him or her immediately to your vet and ask for a test for Valley Fever. The earlier Valley Fever is diagnosed, the better your pet's medical treatment can be. A second test may be necessary a few weeks later, since antibodies to Valley Fever may not be immediately detectable. See our Testing and Diagnosis Chapter for more information, as most of the information that applies to humans also applies to animals.

Some pets will need the same types of antifungal treatment that is given to humans. Dosages will be different, depending on the size of the animal, but amphotericin B, fluconazole, itraconazole, and the others in our Drugs and Treatment Chapter are used. It is estimated that 85% of dogs with Valley Fever are currently treated with fluconazole.[224]

You may wish to call your pet's veterinarian and other veterinarians in your area for suggestions on ways that you can find the medicine for less money. Some suggestions on how to do this for people and animals are included in our Drugs and Treatment Chapter.

A dog owner received drugs from compounding pharmacies and asked us to share a word of caution for others: Her dog had Valley Fever for a very long time with no improvement in symptoms or titers from the compounding pharmacy's drugs. Later, when she purchased the same prescription from traditional pharmacies (just to see if "people's drugs" would make a difference), her dogs' symptoms and titers both improved almost immediately. This implied that the compounding pharmacy either did not provide the correct dose or the correct drug. We cannot know for sure.

Please be sure you investigate the source of your animal's drugs. If you purchase drugs from a compounding pharmacy and your dog is not improving, you may wish to switch to a traditional pharmacy to see if that makes a difference. Naturally, this does not say all compounding pharmacies will give the wrong drugs or doses, or even that this is what had actually occurred in this instance. Valley Fever is, after all, fairly unpredictable. Still, it is worthwhile to take this into consideration.

Statistics

Epidemiology, the scientific study of how and where disease outbreaks occur, has rarely been applied to Valley Fever in dogs. One study was performed by Dr. Lisa Shubitz in Arizona and was supported by the Valley Fever Vaccine Project of the Americas to assist in statistical analysis. It revealed the following data:[226]

- There is a 28% chance of a dog raised from birth in either Maricopa or Pima County to be infected with Valley Fever by the time he or she is only two years old.
- There is an 11% probability of infection within the first year of life.
- There is a 17% probability of infection within their second year of life.
- It is estimated that 4% of dogs will become ill with Valley Fever annually.

Occurrences in Other Animals

Please note that Valley Fever attacks cats as well. We have received many reports from cat owners that are devastated that their beloved cat contracted this disease. Just as dogs have bone and joint symptoms more frequently, cats also tend to have specific symptoms more often: They suffer skin lesions as the most common form of dissemination. When dissemination attacks the brain in both dogs and cats, it tends to do so as a lesion rather than meningitis (although meningitis and spinal cord infections are still reported and may cause paralysis or death). Dogs typically experience seizures as a result of brain lesions but "cats appear to have a wider range of manifestations, including incoordination, hyperesthesia, seizures, and behavior changes."[224]

Many people misguidedly believe that cats do not contract Valley Fever or get very sick from it. Since most pets are regarded as family members, losing a cat, dog, or any other pet due to Valley Fever is devastating to the whole family.

There is currently an epidemic in dogs in Arizona, and cats also suffer greatly, but Valley Fever can infect any mammal with devastating consequences. The long list of animals that have suffered with this disease includes cattle, horses, llamas, mountain lions, armadillos, and others.

Zoos have been notorious for bringing animals into the endemic regions only to have them contract Valley Fever, and then suffer and die from it. Zoos have brought polar bears, gorillas, chimpanzees, and other animals into the endemic areas and witnessed them becoming infected and frequently dying from Valley Fever's most severe symptoms. Even sea otters have been infected and killed by *Coccidioides* spores blown from California's coast.

Although infection in mammals is very common, it was even found in cold-blooded lizards, such as a Sonoran Lyre Snake at the Phoenix Zoo, and a Sonoran Gopher Snake that died in captivity in Western Oregon. The Gopher Snake was believed either to have been brought through the Southwest or it encountered fomites from endemic areas.[206]

All mammals can contract Valley Fever. Valley Fever disseminates very often in infected dogs and many more cats are being diagnosed now than in the past. To date, there have not been any reported cases of Valley Fever in birds.

Stories of Animals with Valley Fever

Our upcoming comprehensive book on Valley Fever and its history will have much more detailed in-depth information on Valley Fever in all animals, in addition to more stories from pet owners. We hope the sampling of stories below will help readers understand just how devastating Valley Fever can be to the animals that are infected and the people who care about them. Where possible, we provided more information about the animal.

Larsyn, a German Wirehaired Pointer
Age: 1year, 8 months
Home: Bemidji, MN (born Tucson, AZ contracted VF at 4 months)
Owner: Nicole L.

Larsyn was born in Tucson and only lived there for about four months before I moved to MN in October 2005. She developed nasal symptoms in December and then over the course of the next few months I noticed her head was becoming pointy. She had started becoming very lethargic and anorexic. She had lost quite a bit of weight.

I took her to the vet in Bemidji and after he x-rayed her head and gave her IV fluids, my vet recommended I take her to the University of MN Veterinary Hospital for further tests. To my surprise she had Valley Fever. I hadn't known that it could go into the bones, otherwise I would have suggested that test initially since I had lost my first dog, a four year old Boxer four months after moving to Tucson.

Within two weeks on the medicine Larsyn was acting like a new dog. Her titer has gone from a 1:8 to a 1:16 despite daily Itraconazole. She was eating and playing with her toys that for months laid untouched. She even gets excited to take her pill now. We still have a few tests that are not quite normal. Her platelet levels are low and recently her reticulocytes were very high. She has a very high, spoiled quality of life even though she is still fighting this illness. She seems to be a fighter, but I am still nervous that this disease will take away another wonderful dog.

Keisha Carat Love, a Siberian Husky
Age: 8 years
Home: Placentia, CA
Owner: Monica D.

In April 1999, Keisha was a 10 week old female Siberian Husky puppy and we lived in Rhode Island. Later in 1999, Keisha moved with us to Orange County, California. Keisha was always a rambunctious and mischievous puppy, full of energy and vigor. She vocalized, as a Siberian Husky will do, and would demand to be walked or included in family activities.

In August 2000, Keisha moved with me to Chandler, Arizona. We lived there during the academic year and then she spent the summers in Orange County, California. During those years (2000-2002), Keisha still acted with a pleasant disposition, demanding walks and exercise. The dog parks in Tempe, AZ and Chandler, AZ were her favorite daily destination.

During Fall 2002, I initially noticed that Keisha, who had always had fussy eating habits, was not eating regularly at all. I switched dog foods and started to prepare her hamburger meat. She would eat sparingly, but since she still demanded exercise, I attributed her condition to the fact that she was experiencing separation anxiety as I was away from home for much of the day.

In January 2003, we permanently relocated to Orange County, CA. Being around more family members seemed to make Keisha happier and despite my worries about her weight, she had a healthy vet checkup with Dr. C and updated vaccinations in August 2003 in preparation for the arrival of a young Siberian Husky female we rescued.

Around December 2003, Keisha lost interest in eating and would lie down on her stomach to eat her food. She also was snippy towards our other Husky. She no longer wanted to play with her.

In January 2004, a month away from turning five years old, I noticed Keisha yelp when bending her head down to sniff the ground. I thought she may have hurt herself with rough play with our other dog, but her weight, too, was very low. I made a vet appointment with Dr. Y and was accused of neglect since Keisha was down to 33 pounds. However, Keisha's "normal" weight was never more than 40 pounds.

Dr. Y took x-rays of Keisha and determined that Keisha's painful neck was most likely the result of a slipped disk in her neck. She put her on Prednisone and for a week, we noticed that Keisha wanted to eat and play again. About 8 days later, though, Keisha suddenly began to yelp, pant, and pace. I was going to wait for her check up the following day, but Keisha looked dazed and seemed to be losing her ability to walk.

By the time I reached Dr. Y's office, Keisha was trembling and losing her ability to walk and her breathing was very labored. Dr. Y immediately referred us to Dr. Hanson, in Tustin, CA. He took x-rays, did a dye test to see where her spinal cord was affected and performed emergency surgery to remove a tumor (near the middle of her back) that was pinching her spinal cord. Without the surgery, Keisha would have died within a short time.

Dr. Hanson was able to determine from the blood work, the type of gelatinous tumor, and Keisha's personal history (having lived and played in Chandler, Arizona) that Keisha had Valley Fever. After surviving and working through the surgery on her spine, Keisha began taking Ketoconazole for the Valley Fever.

Ketoconazole was a nightmare medication for us. Keisha would refuse to eat, appeared nauseous and didn't have much energy. We had to figure out a small pocket of time after she'd get her dose of Prednisone (for her back) where she'd actually want to eat and then my brother, who she trusted not to give her medication, would hand feed her rice balls with peanut butter, or Science Diet canned food mixed with hamburger meat. We had to continuously monitor Keisha's reaction to the Ketoconazole. She developed fatty deposits on her eyes and lost much of her hair. It appeared that the medicine or the illness was affecting her thyroid.

After about 9 months, Dr. Hanson switched Keisha to Fluconazole (Diflucan). It was very expensive. Over $140 for a month supply. After several months we began purchasing from Dr. Foster and Smith and the price went down to less than $30 for a month supply.

On the Fluconazole we noticed marked improvement with Keisha's eating habits and energy levels. With the exception of a few weeks, Keisha was on Fluconazole continuously for over a year. Her energy level returned and except for slight neurological damage to her rear leg (from the tumor), Keisha has been able to run and play as normal.

Fall 2006, Keisha discontinued Fluconazole and seemed to thrive. Her coat was full and thick. She reached 41 pounds and enjoyed playing and going for brisk walks.

Recently, as of February 2007, Keisha began to act bored/depressed as we were not walking her regularly and around March 20 we noticed Keisha's appetite decrease. During the weekend, Keisha enjoyed a run at the park, but we noticed her panting inappropriately throughout the day and licking her front limbs and genital area. We have made an appointment with Dr. Hanson to test her titer levels, as her condition seems to get a little worse everyday (she is restless and will not eat unless forced).

Valley Fever has been a horrible disease for our pet. Without much intervention and expensive medical procedures, medicine, time consuming rehabilitation, and a tremendous amount of support and love, Keisha would not have come this far. Our hope and wish is that pet owners are made aware of this disease so that they can be spared from its effects.

Boots, a Boxer/Pit Bull
Age: 16 months
Home: Mojave, CA (infected in Barstow, CA)
Owner: Cheryle Hatcher

Boots does not want to eat, vomits, has Grand Mal seizures, major weight loss, loss of motor skills (equilibrium, walking, barking and hearing loss at times), 24 hours a day eyes are draining mucus, sleeps 21 out of 24 hours a day and just plain lifeless.

I have spent about $9,500 to date on keeping my son (pet) alive. None of the meds from the vet have helped him so I decided to treat him like I raised him: "Human store bought items and over the border (Mexican) meds and a lot of TLC along with 24 hour care." He has had all the following symptoms: cough, weight loss, lack of appetite, fever, depression, malaise, wheezing, lameness, sudden seizures, swollen joints, skin abscesses and change in personality.

We take each day as a blessing. Boots could be running and playing being normal one day and the next day being close to death. Everyone wanted me to put him down because he was suffering and he was, but I have a lot of love and patience. I refused to give up on him. He still isn't through or at a point where I can leave him alone. If he isn't with me I have a babysitter. Boots has had a change in personality. He has become a very mean dog. He has bitten someone he has been raised around so I don't trust him around anyone anymore. I have to keep a close eye on him when there is anyone around. He has even nipped at me.

Before VF he was full of life, lots of energy, love and kindness and very healthy. After VF he is mean, lifeless, no energy, sad, depressed, has bad seizures, problems with hearing and blindness.

December 2007 Update:

Cheryle told me that if it wasn't for the night vet that she saw when Boots was taken in to the hospital to begin with he might not have been diagnosed properly. That particular vet's wife had Valley Fever and he was very familiar with the signs and symptoms because of that.

Boots is doing better. The seizures have stopped, he has gained weight and is happy. He coughs a lot if he tries to run and his muscles hurt sometimes not allowing him to walk on one of his legs, but all in all Cheryle is grateful that Boots is still with her.

Loki (deceased)
Age: 7 yrs
Home: Tucson, AZ
Owner: Georgette R.

Loki was on Fluconazole. She experienced weight loss, loss of appetite, malaise, a change in personality and depression. Before contracting VF, Loki led an active lifestyle. She played fetch with a tennis ball daily, was very perky and healthy prior to her Valley Fever illness. Loki passed away from VF.

Bernadette, a German Shepherd Mix (deceased)
Age: 8-9 months old (stray)
Home: Mesa (infected Apache Junction) AZ
Owner: Brooke S.

I found this dog on the streets. She was lame, skinny and covered in sores. Since I have had her she has put on weight, though I sometimes have to forcefeed her. Her sores are getting worse. Hopefully the meds will help after she has been on them a little longer. When I found her she had a cough, diarrhea, was very thin, didn't want to eat, a fever, swollen joints and was lame.

The vet recommended amputation of her lame leg. Bernadette is expected to be on meds for at least one year.

Bernadette died on December 15, 2006. Valley Fever had disseminated into her bones and she had sores all over the pads of her feet. She died of kidney failure, which Brooke said was from the medication for her VF.

Rocky, a Rottweiler
Age: 8 yrs
Home: Peoria, AZ
Owner: Dianne S.

I can't really tell if Rocky has any medication side effects since his VF symptoms are so many. Rocky has swollen joints, lameness and weight loss. He has been on Fluconazole but his prognosis is not very good. He is getting worse each day. Rocky can barely get around. It is hard for him to eat and go outside a few times a day. He can't bear weight on his right front leg and has no feeling in it. The tumor in his head is getting larger. Rocky will most likely never recover. His chances are very slim. He is in constant pain even with the medication. We will have to make a decision soon about putting him down.

Before VF Rocky was a great active family dog. He loved to go for rides and spend time in the outdoors. He was a wonderful pet and great watchdog. We have had Rocky since he was a pup and he has grown up with our children. He loved to play hide and seek.

Riley, a Labrador Retriever
Age: 3.5 years
Home: Phoenix, AZ
Owner: Charles E.

There were no overt symptoms until she had a seizure. Her temperature was 106 and she also had lameness. It took the emergency vet five days to finally diagnose her with Valley Fever. Riley has slowed down quite a lot, is still mildly active but has numerous medical problems due to contracting Valley Fever. She has to be on medication (Fluconazole) for the rest of her life due to the dissemination throughout her organs at the time of diagnosis.

Flick, an English Setter
Age: 7 yrs
Home: Lake Havasu City, AZ
Owner: Margaret D.

Flick had sudden seizures, swollen joints, skin abscesses and lameness all with a 1:8 titer. We are only two weeks into this disease and I never got a prognosis from the vet. My dog is on phenobarbital and is still seizing.

This was a very active English Setter that I exercised every night by walking two miles. He had some intermittent lameness and before we could get him in to see the vet he went into full grand mal seizures. It took a lot of medication to break the seizure activity. It has been a long two weeks and tonight he had another seizure. I feel that his prognosis is probably not promising at this point. Flick certainly does not have quality of life right now.

Lena, a black and tan Coonhound (deceased)
Age: 3 months when diagnosed
Home: Phoenix, AZ
Owner: Debbie O.

I am Lena's third owner; I rescued her. She has been seen by 2 vets with the previous owner, and 2 vets with me. We recently changed vets for the VF because her titers were not coming down and the VF has disseminated into several bones, including her right hip.

She appeared to be a normal healthy pup at adoption in July 2005. Shortly thereafter she began complaining of pain in front legs with limping. By September she developed skin lesions. Her pain has improved, but she still limps with over exertion and can't go on walks anymore. Her titers are still 1:256 and her last two titers were 1:256 as well. At least she has normal growth and development, and her life is pretty good compared to most, but not what it would be without the VF. I suspect it will get a whole lot worse if I don't get this turned around ASAP.

Debbie had updated Lena's story.

Sadly Lena lost her battle with VF on December 6, 2006. We attempted the Abelcet (Amphotericin with Lipid Complex) and had consulted extensively with the VFCE in Tucson. The extra expense incurred was a little over $3000 (in addition to what we had already spent). We could have spent a million, and it wouldn't have mattered...tissue samples were sent to the University of Alabama and the VF had disseminated to all her organs.

Unbelievable...all that medication and it barely slowed it down. Some say we were really lucky that she should have died a long time ago. She was only 18 months old when she died. I miss her terribly. She had open, weeping wounds at the end of her treatment so we are just praying our other five dogs don't get sick.

Lena was not the only part of Debbie's family to be affected by Valley Fever.

I have had Valley Fever 3 times since living in Arizona. The last two times were really frustrating as the docs were condescending during the last two episodes and stated most emphatically that Valley Fever could only be contracted once, so I could not possibly have had it on a previous diagnosis. They all thought the previous docs had misdiagnosed my illness.

I suspect that I may have had a 4th undiagnosed occurrence. I was sent to a University of Arizona infectious disease doc, but they never could diagnosis my swollen lymph nodes from my head to my groin and the skin lesions, and the severe fatigue. They did not even consider a Valley Fever recurrence since I had "already had it." They were thinking in terms of measles, but all their tests came back negative, except to show that I had some sort of infection.

Sadly, my brother has lost two of the lobes of his right lung to Valley Fever. The lobes were removed in 2 separate surgeries that were about 5 years apart, due to VF. The last time his lung collapsed and he almost died from the infection. He is now disabled. It has been about 20 years since his last occurrence.

It was very kind of you to send the link for www.imom.org. *Very much appreciate it. I have been very blessed so far, and have been able to keep pace with her medical bills. But it is good to know that if there should be a need, I have options. Also it is good to know that I can donate to help another that is not as fortunate as I am.*

I read your mom's story. Heartbreaking. [eds: Although a brief version of Sharon's story appears on the web site, David and Sharon both answer e-mails.] *My prayers go out for her. There's nothing that I can add that you all don't already know about Arizona's laissez faire attitude with the disease. Thanks for taking the initiative on this. It is rare that we hear about how this disease affects our visitors.*

Gizmo, a Shih Tzu
Age: 2 yrs
Home: Mesa, AZ
Owner: Boni H.

Gizmo has been taking Fluconazole for five months and she had a mild lack of appetite just when the drug was given, so I feed her first. She then had no problem eating. She started with respiratory problems. When she got excited she would stop breathing. I gave her resuscitation and took her immediately to my doctor.

They thought it was Valley Fever and Gizmo had an X-ray and blood tests that confirmed VF. After that she started to have constant coughing. In the beginning I revived her more than 13 times and then the cough seemed to replace those times she would stop breathing altogether.

I took her to a very good hospital here and the internists decided to try prednisone for a while to stop the cough. Two days before I started the dose she stopped coughing and was suddenly her old self again. She was playing with toys which she hadn't done in five months. She would have some good days and I would think she was getting well. The next day or so she would be sleeping most of the day. We did give her the prednisone for a short period of time with decreasing doses and now she is off that.

Her coughing has come back in brief episodes where I have to give her hydrocc. Every six hours. Now for the last five days she has had diarrhea which she has never had before. I feed her a lot of chicken anyway along with royal canine Shih Tzu food.

I am in my sixth month of constant care. I love her to death and will do anything for her but this disease is so frustrating. I am on disability and work a few days a week. My house is up for sale as I have to downsize to be able to meet my bills. For the last five months I have been sleeping on the couch with her day and night.

Barkley, a Golden Retriever
Age: 18 months
Home: Scottsdale, AZ
Owner: Kelly W.

He was a typical ten month old Golden puppy. Extremely playful and loved to run and play with anyone. Now he cannot run or play with other dogs. Any time he plays hard he seems to get really sick again.

Barkley was off medication for two months. He got extremely ill again and could not walk. On the medication again...stronger dose but titer count is really low and the vet is even confused. The medication does not seem to be working as quickly as it did the first time.

Simon, a Boxer
Age: 2 years
Home: Phoenix, AZ
Owner: Lori S.

I do Boxer rescue in Arizona and we have taken in four VF dogs so far in 2007! Titers ranged from 1:4 to 1:256. Simon's titer was a 1:256. All dogs had muscle atrophy and lameness. All dogs came from the pound and were scheduled to be euthanized due to health status. Three dogs have bone lesions but all are progressing and one is now able to walk on all four legs!

We are doing all that we can to educate the public about this disease in our pets and that it is NOT a life sentence. Fry's carries a VERY inexpensive fluconazole that runs about $10.00 a month for my rescues.

Greta, a Weimaraner
Age: 8 years
Home: Brule, Wisconsin (contracted VF in Tubac, AZ)
Owner: Cate Van Lone-Taylor

Greta has been on Fluconazole for one month so far. She exhibited lameness, swollen joints and a change in personality. She has a lesion in her right hip and lower left leg. I am praying her prognosis is very good. Greta was a very active, very happy and extremely loving dog prior to VF.

December 2007 Update

Even though Valley Fever had disseminated to her bones, the fluconazole has enabled Greta to stop limping and she is now living a relatively normal life. Cate hopes it continues to stay that way.

Jessie, a Balinese Cat (deceased)
Age: 10 months
Home: Pleasant Hill, CA (purchased from breeder in Tucson AZ)
Owner: Marilyn D.

We purchased Jessie from a fabulous Balinese cat breeder in Tucson, Arizona. He was a loving, sensitive beautiful kitten. One month after bringing Jessie home he developed a detached retina. Our vet sent us to the University of Davis Vet Hospital where we worked with three specialists. They tried so hard to save his precious life. After the team of vets solved the mystery of Valley Fever (we have not seen it here) Jessie was too weak to fight. Jessie died three months after diagnosis. He was only ten months old.

Sehnsational Summer Storm, a Bengal Cat (deceased)
Age: 4.6 yrs
Home: Tucson, AZ
Owner: Susan S.

She was a breeding cat and had kittens born a little less than two months before her death. Her symptoms were weight loss and sudden seizures. She was put down because she was too sick.

Sehnsational Agnij, a Bengal Cat
Age: 4 years
Home: Tucson, Arizona
Owner: Susan S.

Agnij' symptoms were depression, lameness and change in personality. His titer was a 1:64. He has been on Fluconazole for four months.
Agnij was nearly paralyzed. His T2 vertebrae was half destroyed by the organism and swelling and inflammation caused him pain and weakness. He is the only male kitten I kept in my breeding program out of Sehnsational Summer Storm (Rani) the cat I reported died of VF on January 15, 2007.

Agnij was chosen to stay with me as a pedigreed stud in my Bengal breeding program.   He did not father any living kittens and had been neutered. He is now a beloved pet but he is so strong (the muscles of his neck are so well developed) that it is really hard to give him his medicines!

Stories from Valley Fever Survivors

It is easy for family members, co-workers, and friends to dismiss concerns about this disease when they don't understand what it can mean to become infected with Valley Fever. It has been estimated that 3-10% of the population that lives in endemic zones inhales *Coccidioides* spp. spores each year. This does not include national and international visitors who unwittingly take this disease home with them. We hope this book demonstrates the seriousness of this disease.

There were 5,535 provisional diagnoses reported in Arizona in 2006. Even before the year was half over, it was clear that the state's Department of Health Services knew to expect yet another record breaking year of Valley Fever infections and admitted this to local newspapers.

> "State health officials have seen such an increase in valley fever cases in early 2006 that state epidemiologist David Engelthaler is calling this 'the year of the spore.'"[81]

Since only 2% of the total overall infections are believed to be diagnosed accurately, the full estimate of Valley Fever infections in Arizona for 2006 is over 276,000. This number is *staggering*. The national number of cases reported to the CDC was 8,916. The estimated national total is over 445,000 people. 2007 was nearly as bad.

Remember once you contract Valley Fever the infection is permanent and there is no cure. This disease can and has activated many times in people even decades after the initial infection, causing their demise.

I hope you will read the stories of those that have contracted Valley Fever and their families. These will give you a glimpse into the disastrous effect it can have on a persons' health, their family, their livelihood, and their future.

Survivors In Their Own Words...

Debi E.
Porterville, California
Contracted VF at age 41

I too am a VF survivor, but just barely, because I continue to suffer from the residual effects of the disease. My entire way of life changed, seemingly overnight. I was very physically active, healthy, fiercely independent and quite capable of caring for myself my entire life. I was in the process of fixing up my house to sell and "move up," since I had recently received a promotion. Everything stopped....plans, dreams, goals, my music, and other hobbies.

I was infected five years ago and have been disabled from a job I worked at for nearly 30 years. I was infected on a construction site and was medically retired out of my job, because I was no longer strong enough or healthy enough to continue. I am still fighting for compensation for it. They took care of me initially, but hurriedly pushed me back to work when I was still ill and I haven't been the same since. They abandoned me, saying that what I have now has nothing to do with VF, even though I was never sick before the VF.

They say I now have Fibromyalgia/Chronic Fatigue Syndrome which boils down to "chronically sore and stiff muscles and never-ending fatigue." Just exactly the way I felt when I first became infected with VF....hmmmm. I've coined the phrase, "Post Valley Fever Syndrome," because I know of many others who after suffering a bout with VF, have ended up with the same diagnoses as me, but the doctors refuse to listen.

I now have to have help with just about everything; laundry, cooking, driving, grocery shopping, paying bills, cleaning house, etc. What friends or family won't help me with, I have to pay for, such as lawn and yard care, which I always preferred to do myself, before being stricken down with Valley Fever.

I'm mostly housebound now. It's very difficult to keep social contacts and appointments, due to all of the doctor appointments, tests for this, tests for that and the debilitating fatigue that can come upon you without much warning....and of course, the excruciating, ever present, relentless pain and burning in just about every muscle and joint in my body. This pain has been here for almost 5 years. It began about a week before I came down with pneumonia caused by coccidioidomycosis. The intensity of the pain waxes and wanes, but there's never a day or night that it's not with me. Loss of my independence and vitality is the greatest loss of all due to Valley Fever and it doesn't look as though I'm going to get it back 100% anytime soon. That's been my highest cost.

I felt the need to write about my experiences with this horrible disease and how it has negatively affected just about every area of my life and the lives of others whom I've talked to about their experiences and outcomes with VF . But I've had to focus my energies on trying to recover from this illness and just get through each day, one day at a time.

The toll that VF takes on one's life is not only financial. In my experience with the disease, it has taken away my ability to think clearly, to be as independent as I have always been, my ability to work (I was gainfully employed at the same institution for 26 years), and the bubbly energy that I once had has also been taken away.

Sharon, I applaud you in this endeavor. I'm very excited that you have the energy and drive to do the studying, writing and research to bring awareness to and shine as much light on the topic of VF as possible. The real lack of information out there is actually appalling for such a dangerous disease that affects just about everyone in different ways.

It has to start somewhere....you're the first ripple in a huge, still pond. Thank you for giving the victims of Valley Fever a voice. Best of luck to you!

Tom Horel (deceased)
Written by Glen and Leslie K. in Kelowna, B.C.
Tom contracted VF in Mesa, AZ

My mother and father in-law couldn't have been more excited about their new retirement home in Mesa at one of the newer mobile home parks. They had purchased their park model in the fall of 1992 and were looking forward to spending their winters in the heat. Tom Horel just turned 70 and was the specimen of perfect health. A scratch golfer, avid swimmer, could whip my butt at squash or racquetball (I was 38) and just an all around athlete.

Tom and Shirley decided to put in a patio in the back yard. After a few days of digging in the sand, he had developed a severe rash and noticed he had some problems breathing. Being a person who rarely had the need to visit a doctor, he decided to ignore the symptoms, not knowing anything about the dreaded "Valley Fever." After a few days, his breathing progressively got worse to the point where he had to be hospitalized. The original diagnosis was pneumonia and after a few days of declining health, they diagnosed Tom with Valley Fever.

The disease had already attacked his lungs, kidneys and was rapidly spreading throughout his body. Within two weeks he was gone leaving a devastated family searching for answers. As time went on we began to get more information about the "best kept secret in North America!"

Nicole G.'s story via e-mail

What scares me about Valley Fever is how little doctors know about the disease. I went to a doctor due to extreme difficulty breathing, chest pains and fatigue and swelling of my joints. I saw a doctor who gave me a breathing treatment and sent me back to work. That night I went to urgent care and saw a different doctor at a different location who told me "not to worry, you have an allergy to something."

I went back two weeks later and was diagnosed with walking pneumonia. In all I went to the doctors five times in six months and saw four different doctors. It was only when my regular doctor (who I had never seen for these issues) looked at my latest X-rays and saw the nodule in my lung. This was the same nodule that had been there since February this year. The same nodule that none of the other four doctors thought to be too concerned about.

I thank God she looked at that X-ray or I would still be getting dramatically worse. I have a case of disseminated cocci and I am angry that none of these doctors saw or were concerned enough to look into my illness more. I can only think there are people who probably still do not know. Thank you for your web site. It has helped me.

Robert Burchfield
Contracted VF at 27 years old in the Lemoore, CA area
Atlanta, GA

I had 3 surgeries of the lung before the diagnosis was VF. I was extremely sick to the stomach, lost 50 pounds in less than 2 months, had lung surgery 3 separate times in less than 2 weeks due to recurring bouts of pneumonia with no signs of letting up. At one point my family was told my chances of surviving until the weekend were not too promising (this was on Wednesday). And had not a visiting doctor, Dr. Wennberger from the CDC, overheard a couple of interns discussing my symptoms while eating lunch, I most likely wouldn't be sitting here now.

Amphotericin B was used to control it last time, not something I would wish on my worst enemy. Well, maybe a couple of treatments, but certainly not daily for four months, then only twice a week for the next two. That's some nasty stuff.

Ever since my Valley Fever infection 16 years ago, it seems life has been a never-ending battle fighting off the cold, flu, and bouts of pneumonia. My scars hurt whenever a cold front is coming. Just recently fungal skin lesions have appeared at the facial area, spreading quickly to the sinus region, temples, lymph nodes.

My initial medical bills pretty much wiped my wife and I out, even with the insurance. Doctor bills alone were over $750,000. Added to the hospital cost and it went well over a million. My company's insurance dropped me from coverage at diagnosis, as it was a pre-existing illness (only been there little over a year after leaving the military). They then turned around and billed me for everything they had paid (only a quarter million then). The VA wouldn't hear anything about it, claiming the lack of any proof (4 years of living just outside of Fresno California, dead in the middle of the valley be damned).

Naturally I lost my job after 49 days of being in intensive care, next was both new cars, then the house. Bankruptcy was the only way to fight off the hospital costs in order to continue treatment, till it got down to having to send our three kids to live with relatives or starve them to death.

I had absolutely no energy after surgery and the medication to combat VF was worse than can be imagined. It took a little over three years to get back on my feet, obtain full time employment, couple years later we bought another house (fixer upper that has tripled in price since then), plus my wife and I will celebrate our 31st wedding anniversary in a couple of months.

So, 16 years after and still kicking. I believe I can live with that. Presently, the half dozen (today anyway) lesions on my face are about the size of a quarter, most joined together by swollen canals just beneath the surface of the skin. Small children can't help but stare, and it can be a nasty mess when the "dam" bursts, but what a relief on the old head bone. The headaches can get to be a bit much, and I can't stress "much" hard enough to get my point across being as I've only been prescribed your basic over the counter pain relievers.

Some days I can go through a 10 pack of BC Powders by early afternoon with only minor relief until it gets to the point all I can do is sit quietly in a darken room listening to my stomach eat a hole in itself. [eds: This over-the-counter pain medication can harm the stomach.]

How long I hold out each day depends on the amount of light and the noise level I put myself into and I'll have to admit there are times those lesions may need a little assistance in getting started in draining.

Bright lights seem to bring on the headaches much faster, after which sounds become more intense. I've been told that what I am describing is exactly how a person who suffers from migraines would describe one of their attacks, but that theirs may last for days. I don't see how those poor folks can handle it.

If I control the lights and noise mine will ease up within an hour or two. But if I can't, like when traveling—especially air travel, it's like someone taking a chainsaw to your head and even little sounds are like thunder. I would imagine it looks pretty strange too, some nut with knuckles buried into his temples, eyes all squelched tight, that jumps every couple of seconds like he'd just been shot.

May be hard to clarify the facts behind it all being that the Doc says basically this is all in my head. Sorry, cheap attempt towards humor, but that's where all major efforts are being directed at the moment.

I want a few better answers about why my knees seem to give out and the over all loss of stamina within just the last couple of months. I think the doctors have a case of tunnel vision themselves and are only looking at the lesions covering the facial area.

Robert provided a follow-up later.

I fired my VF "specialists" and they're to stay fired unless my current doctor says otherwise. If he says they'll have to stay or I'd go without their care, I don't see how going without would be to my long-term disadvantage anyway.

Those clowns made it sound as if I had no idea what I was talking about when I asked about my symptoms, didn't bother to even look over any of the information I'd prepared, and worst, not a single one could give me the three primary areas that are normally targeted by disseminated cocci (although the lab tech guy did get two correct). [Eds: Incidentally, the most common sites of dissemination are the skin, bones/joints, and meninges.] The doctors acted offended that I should even question their abilities, then regrouped into an arrogant bunch wanting to inform me that I was mistaken to think of Valley Fever seriously.

That would be right about when I told them they were fired. They didn't believe me at first, looked somewhat shocked really, until I added a few explicates to show just how fired they really were. Then reality kicked in big time. Not much was said to me while I gathered my things, not directed to me anyway.

Fred D.
Lexington, Maine
Contracted VF at age 48 in Tucson, AZ.

My parents lived in Tucson and both died in 2001. I was in Tucson about a dozen times in 2001. My last visit was to prepare their house for sale. I must have inhaled a big dose of cocci spores. I first felt symptoms in late January 2002. I got progressively worse in February to the point where I needed hospitalization. It wasn't until I had a lymph node biopsy that a positive diagnosis was made. When VF returned in August 2002 I had a very difficult time convincing doctors that it was indeed the cocci. They said there was no way that a person with a healthy immune system could see the cocci come back...but it was. Fortunately, they restarted the Itraconazole soon enough so the symptoms never got really bad again. I'll always be looking over my shoulder for those cocci spores. I can't ever imagine returning to Arizona! It's been a huge ordeal.

Toni C.
Bakersfield, California
Contracted VF at age 35

VF changed the quality of my life. I have trouble staying healthy for a prolonged period of time. It has severely curtailed my abilities physically which has caused problems with jobs, hobbies, etc. I ended up being told by my MD to quit my teaching position. It angers me that in an endemic area such as Bakersfield, MDs don't routinely test for VF in the presence of obvious symptoms.

I know of three people who have been diagnosed with the moderate to meningitis form of Valley Fever only after I recommended they request the tests from their doctors. Can you imagine? A young woman, pregnant, black no less with symptoms for her entire pregnancy, not being tested? [Eds: It is well documented that black Valley Fever patients are at an increased risk for dissemination and death.] *She had to collapse and end up with shunts, surgeries, etc...it's criminal to subject people to medical care from physicians with blinders on...people die from this disease, have their whole lives changed, and still it is ignored. I hate having to say "I can't do that anymore" and I'm only 47.*

Charles R.
Dallas, Texas
Contracted VF at age 36 in Phoenix, Arizona

I have celiac disease (CD). CD is an inherited autoimmune condition wherein, if one eats wheat, rye, oats or barley there is an autoimmune reaction that over time depletes the immune system. I had been diagnosed with CD about four months before contracting VF. I have no other known illnesses, particularly of the immune system.

I was forced to drop out of life because of VF. I became very ill. The biggest problem was that doctors couldn't or wouldn't help me. Even in Phoenix where I fell ill, I went to the doctor and was diagnosed with a chest cold and given antibiotics. A few weeks later when I figured out what was wrong (I was still sick) another doctor in Phoenix refused to treat me. His nurse said, "Dr. X doesn't treat VF patients. You'll need to see a specialist." From there it was a nightmare. I have given up calls to physicians. They were far more concerned with my insurance coverage and with their liability than they were with helping the sick.

The Valley Fever Center for Excellence is not very helpful either. The same physicians they have on their referral list also refused to treat me for liability and insurance reasons. I notified the VFCE of this but they made some mealy-mouthed excuse. I told them to spend some time finding doctors who really were willing to treat sick people.

Things became more complicated when I transferred to Dallas last summer. Most of the doctors hadn't heard of VF and weren't interested in a learning curve. I even consulted infectious disease specialists and pulmonologists. Finally I found a general practitioner in Oklahoma City (220 miles from Dallas) who had heard of VF and would treat me.

Last summer the infection disseminated from my lungs. First it went into my intestines causing the most intense cramping and diarrhea that lasted for two days before abating. Then it spread to my meninges causing severe headaches and blurry vision. The whole time I had pustules, rashes on my feet, legs and arms and less frequently on my chest.

Most of my life ended. I had no time or energy for activities. I had to move out of my apartment (breaking the lease) because the apartment was moldy and I can no longer tolerate dampness or mold growth in my living space. I still have relapses of the lung and skin.

Mary Jane S.
Walnut Creek, California
Contracted VF at age 19

I had no major health issues other than a cold about once a year and the flu every few years prior to contracting Valley Fever. When I was first diagnosed I thought I just had the flu and an ear infection. I was a student at UCSB at the time and after several visits to the Student Health Center with no improvement, they finally sent me to the Santa Barbara County Health Department for a VF skin test. It was positive and I was sent home with antibiotics. I only missed a few days of class and felt completely better a few weeks later.

I had a pretty bad flare up of Valley Fever nineteen years (at age 39) after the first symptoms appeared...painful red nodules on my legs, which lasted about eight weeks until fading into flat bruises. There was chest pain and cough. I was only out of work that time a few days, but felt tired for about six weeks. I have had a few mild flare ups since then, but didn't miss work or let it interfere with my everyday life. I didn't give VF another thought until about five years ago.

I noticed several painful nodules begin to appear on my legs. I started coughing and came down with what I believe was a full blown cold. The cough lingered and was accompanied by a pressure in my lungs which I had never felt before. It hurt to breathe. I just felt this pressure like someone was sitting on my chest.

I still get nodules on my legs occasionally. The cough lingers...gets worse upon major exertion, but sometimes flares up even if I'm just sitting quietly.

Valley Fever has been a nagging chronic illness which I can ignore at times, but just when I forget I have it, it all seems to rear its ugly head as a reminder that it exists within me.

It does frighten me to think that it could become much more severe in the future.

Nancy I.
Phoenix, Arizona
Contracted VF at age 48

I lived in Phoenix for more than fifteen years with no problem. I moved to my current location in 1998 where there is constant ongoing construction. I called the county numerous times regarding construction not using adequate dust abatement. I contracted Valley Fever within a year of moving here. So did two of my neighbors. I had to stop my long history of bicycling due to tremendous muscle and joint pain. The diagnosis took a long time because I never had a cough. They tell me the nasal-pharyngeal area was where it started. I still have frequent sinus infections and headaches as well as tire easily.

They are again doing construction and my dog has now contracted the disease. He was diagnosed yesterday. The financial impact for the dog alone is huge and we just received the diagnosis. He has a bone mass— went through a cancer scare and found out it was Valley Fever osteomyelitis.

For construction, they blade acres of land removing all the vegetation and even if some of the responsible builders water while working, it dries and a small breeze can envelope people in dust and dirt. Many builders are irresponsible and I have driven through clouds of dirt they cause when they blade clear acres of desert. Calling county or the builder is ineffective. The problem of construction needs to be addressed.

Fred C.
Bakersfield, California
Contracted VF at age 16

The Amphotericin B treatments caused numerous complications, nausea, weakness, up to grand mall seizures and hospitalizations. VF affected my skin, lungs, spine, eyes, adrenal glands and nose.

I haven't been able to get as far away from Bakersfield as I'd like. After being sick, I wanted to escape to any other part of the country, mostly New York, if for any other reason, to get out of the city that ruined my life. However, because of continual complications, relapses and emergency trips to the hospital, I am realizing that this will probably never happen. I was able to move to Santa Barbara to go to college, but was forced to drop out due to medical issues. In basic terms, I hate Valley Fever and everything it stands for.

Mark S.
Georgetown, Texas
Contracted VF at age 12 or 13 years old in Tucson, AZ

I went on home study for most of the rest of high school. I could not sit for more than 30 minutes at a time due to pain. I still have this problem.

I was rejected for at least three jobs (Douglas Aircraft, Hughes Aircraft and City of Los Angeles) and the military. This was before EEO and during the Vietnam time. When I was 17 I was rejected by the military after signing up for the draft. My parents were happy...I was very depressed. I still am, after 40 years of pain.

I had no health issues prior to VF. After VF I had two surgeries. After the second surgery, the surgeon said that the joint had evidence of coccidioidomycosis infection.

Bernice B (deceased)
Green Valley, Arizona
Contracted VF at age 84

In January 2000 Mom was her vital, wonderful self despite the fact that Dad had been diagnosed with terminal cancer two months earlier and was under hospice care. Her concern for him on top of her own misery once she began vomiting and having extraordinary headaches in early February was difficult, yet her spirit remained wonderful.

The entire family knew that Mom would live beyond Dad barring some very unusual event. Her health was excellent and her attitude even better, despite the limits her arthritis placed on her. Arrangements had been made for the eldest son to help her with financial matters once Dad was gone.

The unusual did happen. Not only did she contract coccidioidomycosis, but it disseminated and was not diagnosed until five days after she went into a coma. She lived in an endemic area and was seeing supposedly excellent doctors who had been practicing in the area for extended periods, etc.

Dad missed Mom terribly during the three and a half months he lived beyond her. They lived good lives and relatively long lives. Yet the Valley Fever experience still haunts me. Mom died on March 30, 2000 from cocci meningitis.

As far as we know, Bernice was not even aware of Valley Fever until she was diagnosed with it. She lived in Arizona for 20 years before she contracted Valley Fever and it tragically took her life.

Martha M.
Macon, Georgia
Contracted VF at age 55

I am still in the early stages of this disease...have to hire a housekeeper to do household chores, go shopping for me and run errands, etc. I no longer am able to attend church or go to any social activities. The pain in joints and muscles are so severe that I can not do a walking regime any longer. Getting in and out of a car is excruciating. Because my immune system is so compromised at this time, I have to avoid crowds to avoid any further infections. My diabetes is worse and I am not responding to my medications. I learned of VF after contracting the disease.

My husband was retired but had to return to full time work as I can not work at present. After we returned from our trip to the Southwest, I got pneumonia and was treated with 3 different antibiotics with no help. My stepdaughter who lives in Surprise, Arizona mentioned that their dog died from VF and so she knew the fungus was in their soil and suggested I be tested.

Corinna N.
Bakersfield, California
Contracted VF at age 26

I was an asthmatic prior to VF. I became sick on February 9, 2003. I had plans for Valentines Day which I wasn't able to do. I thought I had the flu. I went to the doctor and was told I had the flu and asthma problems and was given a breathing treatment. A week later I felt better and returned to the gym only to feel very weak and tired after...suddenly had a high fever. It lasted for a week until I was taking a shower and almost collapsed with a fever of 104.1.

I went to the doctor the next day and they did a chest x-ray and told me I had bronchitis. I believed I had Valley Fever but didn't say anything because I thought the doctors knew more than I did. About a week later I developed a rash that looked like hives all over my body, still had high fevers and breathing problems and intense pain in my chest that I thought I was having a heart attack. I had this pain several times over the next week or so. I still believed I had VF. I went back to the doctor and he said my blood tests were okay but my white blood count was a bit high. I asked to be tested for Valley Fever. The doctor said he didn't think I had VF and that it was probably an allergic reaction to something. He tested me anyway.

At that point, I developed an intense indescribable pain in my ribs on my right side which went up into my shoulder. I had a problem with my insurance and was not able to get my results for 3 weeks. Finally, last week (April 7, 2003) I was diagnosed with Valley Fever. I was told it was unlikely for me to get it because I am white and female. If I hadn't insisted on being tested for it I still wouldn't know what was wrong with me.

The doctor told me my last chest x-ray looked good and there is nothing there and my white blood count isn't that high considering I have VF. I told him about the pain in my ribs and shoulder...he said that VF can move around all over your body in a no big deal kind of way.

I can't lie on my left side as well. Every time I have to cough or sneeze or yawn I have to prepare my body for the pain it causes in my ribs. If I take a deep breath it also hurts a lot. I can no longer function normally on a day to day basis. I have two children, one of which is developmentally disabled. It is so difficult for me to care for them and take care of my house. My fiancée has been cooking and cleaning for the last two months plus working a full time job where he is the boss and has a lot of responsibilities.

I stay at home all the time and I am jealous of people that have "normal" lives. I can't make plans to do anything for I don't even know how long. I planned to go to the beach and wasn't able to do that...I will miss my daughters softball games all summer. This has taken a toll on me and my family and I have only been dealing with this disease for 2 1/2 months. I can't imagine feeling this way for another year or more.

I have read others' stories on the VFS message board and it doesn't sound very promising. Initially I didn't think it was a big deal. I would be sick for a while and then be fine, but after reading what other people have experienced, I am very concerned. When my blood tests were done I had a titer of 1:64.

Karen M.
Duluth, Minnesota but also an "Arizona Snowbird"
Contracted VF at age 51 in Fountain Hills, Arizona

I was diagnosed with bacterial pneumonia in the first week of March 2003. I now believe it was cocci pneumonia. Two months later when we were back in Minnesota, I went to the doctor feeling that the "pneumonia" was not totally gone. They found a "mass" on my left lung. For over three weeks, I thought I had lung cancer (especially since I smoked for many years, but quit a couple of years ago).

A friend of mine mentioned "Valley Fever" to me so I did some reading on it and mentioned it to the doctor when he called to give me the results of the CT scan. He said it didn't look like a benign tumor. When I told him about the cocci fungus and that it can look like lung cancer on an x-ray, he very definitely said "No, that's not it."

So another week and a half waiting to have a biopsy! At least the pathologist during the biopsy knew of the cocci fungus and said he would check for it and that's what it turned out to be.

We bought a winter home in Fountain Hills, Arizona so we are also concerned about going back and what the chances are of breathing in more spores and getting sicker. The nodule is still there and a tiny bit smaller than it was in May.

Rachel
Bakersfield, CA
Contracted VF at age 28

My case took six weeks to diagnose even though I live in one of the most well known areas for Valley Fever. I had about ten chest x-rays done that never did show any signs of infection. Finally, after I had already started to feel better, I developed the "valley fever rash" and was then immediately diagnosed. By then I was pretty bad.

I was put on Diflucan for three months and my titers dropped to 1:4. I was taken off with the drug without any follow up. My regular doctor tested me for VF four months after stopping the Diflucan. My titers rose to 1:16 even though I was feeling fine. At that point I sought out an Infectious Disease specialist. He immediately prescribed Diflucan which I have been on for six months.

After about two months on the meds, I began to experience severe side effects including severe debilitating headaches, dizziness, lack of concentration, moodiness, change in menstrual cycles. My doctor was concerned I had developed meningitis. A pharmacist said that taking Diflucan for such a long period coupled with birth control pills can cause serious side effects. The Diflucan causes the hormones in the birth control pills to intensify greatly, causing my headaches, moodiness, etc. I asked my gynecologist to change my birth control pills to something less potent which did help some. I stopped taking the Diflucan. My side effects have returned due to the adjustment of the hormone levels again. I am still having migraine headaches after three weeks but they do seem to be lessening.

The increase in hormone levels from taking Diflucan was not expected and not discussed with me at all. I had to research for myself what the problem was as well as talking with the pharmacist. For someone sensitive to hormone level changes this could be a very bad experience. I'm not sure if the doctors know enough about this medication and all the possible side effects.

Even after three week off the medication my hair is still falling out. When someone has cancer and is going through chemotherapy everyone knows and understands that their hair will fall out and they have compassion for them. With Valley Fever "it's just some hair"...people don't relate it to you being sick and on medication...they just think you have really ugly hair.

This has changed my life. It has put my thoughts of having children on hold until I am off the medication for a full year. I am a much "slower" person than I was. Things take longer...I need to take naps...I need a lot of sleep much more than the normal person. I could sleep sixteen hours straight and still be tired.

Kelly S.
Lancaster, California
Contracted VF at age 40

I just started back to work after my three children were finally in school full time. I worked for about a year. I soon noticed that I was getting tired during the day more than usual. I convinced myself that it was due to getting older. Every time I caught a cold it took me forever to get over it. Finally I caught a cold that I couldn't get rid of and went to urgent care. They took an x-ray.

I was called the next day and was told it was irregular and needed to take another one. They thought it was an old case of TB and it was nothing to worry about. About a year later I couldn't stop coughing and it was painful in my right lung. It dawned on me that the pain was in the same area as the spot on the x-ray. I went to the doctor and the x-ray led to a CT scan which showed that the cavity in my lung had gotten bigger.

The doctor wanted to know why no one was following my case or running tests. (I have an HMO and can never get in to see my doctor, so I get passed on to a new doctor every time which wasted a lot of time). He ripped my chart apart and gave me copies to keep of all my tests. They all said that I had to be followed closely. I didn't know any of this. None of this was told to me.

I lived with the thought that what I had was probably cancer for about eight months. After much more time wasted, I finally got to a specialist and that was when the serious testing to find out what I had started. I took sputum tests and blood tests which were all negative. I had a lung biopsy which showed positive for Valley Fever. This Friday I have to have a spinal tap to see if it has spread to my nervous system.

How many people are walking around sick, being told there is nothing wrong? I mean, I even had a big cavity show up on my x-ray (which should have been a red flag) and they still did nothing.

I am really angry at this insurance company right now. When I think of what I went through for a year and a half it makes my blood boil. I remember my daughter asking me to take her to the mall and I told her "I don't feel good and I have a headache." She said "you never feel good and always have a headache."

I even had to quit my job. So much emotional stuff could have been avoided. At least now I know something was wrong and it wasn't because of getting older.

I thought I knew about Valley Fever, but now I am finding out how misinformed I really was. About 20 years ago my Mother-in-law contracted VF. She lived in this area all her life. All I knew was that once you had it, you had it forever. I also knew it messed with her diabetes. That was back when they didn't know much about it. They just went in and cut it out of her lung.

I always assumed that VF came from animal droppings out in the desert. I also remember people saying "how can you have caught that, I thought it was under control."

I had no idea it was still around and I thought it was only in the Bakersfield area. For some stupid reason I thought the state was able to contain VF by the way people talked about it, so I never concerned myself with it. I also know that there is not much that can be done about it. The wind blows hard here everyday. It is just a fact of life here.

The reason we live here is the paychecks. My husband makes a really good living in aerospace here. I mean, that's what keeps this valley running.

I think that there are a lot of sick people here and they just don't know why. The health department said the biggest problem in this area is chronic illness. I bet if they checked, most of these people have or have had Valley Fever.

Maybe they don't want people to know because a lot of people would leave and that would cause serious problems for the state. If people start leaving, the state would lose money. I'm starting to have second thoughts about if it was worth it. Everyone keeps telling me that the Valley Fever will get better, but every time I go to the doctor, things just seem to be getting worse. I do know this, until doctors start taking this serious and start looking for it, we'll never know just how many people are sick with VF.

Stacy P.
Phoenix, Arizona
Contracted VF at age 36

I will try to make this as short as possible. I experienced a rash and fever in the beginning leading to a course of breathing problems, weakness, fatigue and over all down and out. I thought I was dying and no one could figure out the problem. The x-rays after 2 1/2 weeks indicated pneumonia so I was put on antibiotics...this did nothing and I continued to get worse. On my last visit to the doctors they stated that they were pretty sure that it was Valley Fever but that the blood test came back negative. She did not prescribe medication and told me that it will get better. It did not! I went to the Emergency Room because I was really thinking I was going to die and my husband was extremely worried. I was an extremely active person, hiking, biking, walking, playing sports and all of that has stopped.

By the time I was put on Diflucan the VF had left a sizeable cavity in my lung. The cavity never went away and I was advised after two years that I should have a thoracotomy done. The operation took place a year ago this past February. The doctors did state at the time that this may not take care of all the problems involved with the VF. This is the worst procedure I have ever been through in all my life. I was in the hospital for six days and continue to feel the effects of the surgery. A recent blood test indicates I still have Valley Fever. My doctor was surprised. I explained to him that I knew I still had it. Having VF is such a different feeling. You can actually feel it, like it is an organism invading your body. I am back on Diflucan. I just wish it would go away!

Ronald B.
Portland, Oregon
Contracted VF at age 12 in Granada Hills, California

The first 3 months I was in isolation because no one knew what I had. Doctors thought whatever I had was contagious so I was unable to be around my brothers and sisters or friends for the first 6 months. I had a tutor for schooling for one year after diagnosis. I was too young to know what other negative affects it had on my family. I had no health issue prior to getting this disease. I now suffer from chronic bronchitis.

Lisa M.
Chicago, Illinois
Contracted VF at age 24 in Tucson, Arizona

I have continuing complications. My Valley Fever disseminated. Amphotericin B caused nausea, bone aches, muscle aches and wound up with a kidney infection during the infusion period. My initial titer was 1:64. I have reoccurring joint stiffness and pain in wrists, chest, fatigue and night sweats. I had nothing wrong with my health prior to Valley Fever.

Jeffrey C.
Magna, Utah
Contracted VF at age 10

We as a family are having a hard time with the fact that we were not notified of the possibility that our son could contract this disease by us traveling to California...It is very hard for us as parents to know that because of a family vacation we have put our 10 year old son's life in jeopardy and unsure of his future to come with the disease.

Thomas S.
Lancaster, California
Contracted VF at age 47 or 48

My infection was discovered in November 2001 in Lancaster, California. Symptoms were barely noticeable at first. Now I have extreme chronic fatigue. I lost approximately $80,000 in wages over the past 18 months of this illness.
Valley Fever has affected my skin, joints and lungs. Sufficed to say, my VF has been a living hell that nearly killed me and has nearly bankrupted my family. The fact that I'm even alive is a blessing that my family and I cherish every day.

Greg J.
Murrieta, California
Contracted VF at age 17—now 44 years old

I was on the high school football team at the time and missed the first half of the season. I had hip replacement surgery which a nurse informed me could have been caused by the Valley Fever. I have had bronchitis quite a lot since contracting VF.

Greg C.
Anaheim, California
Contracted VF at age 29 or 30

I don't remember going in to an endemic area before coming down with Valley Fever. The diagnosis took a long time. The doctors did not know what it was and just gave me massive doses of Ibuprofen. I went to the emergency room a couple of times but they still failed to admit me. It was when I started becoming incoherent then I was finally admitted.

I was started on Amphotericin B treatments intrathecally every other day for a couple of months. It burned as it was injected and caused such a severe headache. Boy was that painful. The side effects of the medicine were extreme nausea, vomiting and dizziness. After those treatments stopped they put me on Diflucan. I now take 200 mg twice daily.

Since I was only married a year before I got the disease, my wife and I wondered if we should have kids. We decided that we should and did. I didn't have many problems until four years ago. I had to have a shunt put into my head because of pressure on my brain. I was getting many headaches and neck stiffness. I thought this was due to pressure at work but it was VF.

One morning I woke up vomiting and feeling like the cocci had come back. We went to the emergency room and they did an MRI. I was sent to a neurologist who installed the shunt. They discovered that there was a lot of pressure in my brain because my cerebrospinal fluid was not draining properly. This was caused by the cocci meningitis. I was out of work for another three months. The pressure in my brain made me feel like I was carsick all the time. I was vomiting and the room was always spinning. It took a while for that to go away.

I haven't noticed any problems since but my neurosurgeon who installed the shunt told me that I had had a minor stroke at the time. He also told me that my pancreas was burned and that cataracts are already developing. He said I will probably also become a diabetic.

I had difficulty getting any kind of life insurance. They won't give me a preferred rate. I continue to take Diflucan and have regular blood tests to see how my liver is doing.

Gerald N.
Tucson, Arizona
Contracted VF at age 8-10

I remember being sick most of the time during my early grade school years. I remember breathing being extremely labored. I am always tired and feverish. It was during the later years in my life that I discovered that it WAS Valley Fever that caused my childhood problems. All of the symptoms I had experienced then and the after affects now are due to that awful fungus. My lungs are scarred to this day. I am still lethargic...joints ache...headaches...I especially experience malaise! I have liver and skin problems. I know I am a Valley Fever Survivor.

Linda O.
Peekskill, New York, formerly Apache Junction, AZ
Contracted VF at age 33

I'm from New York and moved to Arizona in 1987 to "start a new life." Got tired of seeing Christmas lights wrapped around cacti and decided to come home to NY, having no idea that I brought with me this nasty fungus.

About two years ago I started having terrible episodes of coughing up blood. This was very frightening. In NY they first thought it was TB. I was given a test and ordered to stay in the house and not have any contact with anyone. Test results for TB were negative. Next step was a bronchoscopy (horrifying experience!). The Culture was sent to CDC in Atlanta. Finally on the last day of the test the culture grew the cocci fungus. I had a CT scan that showed a 6cm cavity in my upper left lung.

I took Diflucan for about a year. The cavity shrunk to 3cm and I was taken off the medication. I had no symptoms until just this past Sunday so I am back on the anti-fungal drugs.

I had to have surgery to remove part of my lung.

Caraly F.
Chandler, Arizona
Contracted VF at age 32

I was in perfect health prior to VF (nonsmoker, nondrinker, no cold/flu, etc. in 15 years prior). Doctors first misdiagnosed as sudden pneumonia (go figure?) and put me on high level antibiotics, which worsened condition until they took x-rays and blood work two weeks later. The condition turned critical and was rediagnosed as severe Valley Fever, which had since spread to tissue and organs, etc. As a result of diagnosis placed on 7 months of antifungal medications.

Pamela B.
Durango, Colorado
Contracted VF at age 31 in Carefree, Arizona

Valley Fever has induced many changes in my life. I lost 22 months of my son growing up when he was 11/12 years old. I went through a divorce. I can no longer workout regularly in the gym. I can not run for any distance, participate in any physical sports and suffer extreme joint pain on a daily basis. I am constantly calling in to say I will be late for work. I call in sick on an average of 3-6 days a month. I keep a great attitude as one can only hope to do.

Todd N.
Odessa, Texas
Contracted VF at age 40 in Green Valley, Arizona

I have daily severe killer headaches, rash, night sweats, vision problems, malaise, nausea, loss of appetite, muscle aches, chest pain, burning sensation in foot, fever, chills, dizziness, stiff neck, speech problems, memory difficulties and learning difficulties.

I now make it to work but don't get an appropriate amount of work done on most days because I am worn out. I could not and can not as of yet go do the things I or my family wants to do. I can not make trips with our race car team because I can't stay up with the pace. For anyone with this debilitating disease I have total sympathy.

Sydniee S.
Gilbert, Arizona
Contracted VF at age 39

They say I had VF for two years and that it is active now. For two years my doctors had been trying to find out what was wrong with me and thought it was other problems when in fact it was and is Valley Fever.

We have no health insurance and can't get it. This is starting to financially ruin us. We can't afford my medicine so I won't get better. I can't work as I am always out of breath. My family is very upset and scared. My husband doesn't know what to do anymore. He can't find a job that will give us insurance. He is a diabetic so insurance is hard to come by. My mother died of Valley Fever two years ago and I know what she went through...sad to say I will suffer like she did and die. I can't get my meds...had enough money to buy five days worth. At $835.00 a month I can't afford it. I am desperate. I am very sick like others and have been for two years. I can't go to any other doctor as I can't afford it so my family guy will have to do.

Sharon
Peoria, Arizona
Contracted VF at age 31

     I have a cocci lung mass that requires surgery. I've had controlled diabetes (juvenile) without complications since the age of 10. Since contracting Valley Fever I lost my job, my marriage is failing, I am depressed and stressed, I have financial problems and surgery is pending to remove the upper lobe of my left lung. My diabetes is getting harder to keep under control, I have hair loss and my lips are peeling causing extreme self-confidence issues, I have abandoned my hobbies and the person I used to be. Frequently I have loss of hope.

Nadine L.
Friendswood, TX
Contracted VF at 42 years old in Sedona, AZ

     I contracted VF in Feb 2004 while I was attending a seminar in Sedona, AZ. I had flu symptoms within 10 days of returning from Sedona. Even though I sought medical attention right away, I continue to battle this disease. I have been hospitalized for pneumonia and currently have a 4 cm lesion on my right upper lobe. My pulmonary doctor is scheduling a bronchoscopy for this week (for a biopsy). I have had the following symptoms since contracting VF.

Flu like symptoms
Night jerks with sleeping and/or end of day
Severe shortness of breath with everyday activity
Chest pain
Severe joint pain (day to day) with "hot" joints
Fever at night
Night Sweats
Nose bleeds
Rash on neck, shoulders and back
Heart Palpitations
Leg weakness and gait disorder
Fatigue

     I have already spent thousands on my medical care, since my doctors had a problem diagnosing me.
     I was very healthy and work as an Occupational Therapist—which has been very physically demanding since contracting VF. I'm a 42 year old white female, who went mountain climbing while visiting Sedona. It was windy and cold and had rained a few days previous to that day. I had no health problems before visiting Sedona, and have had constant health problems since returning from my AZ work related course.
     I am considering legal action against the state of AZ. The world needs to know about this horrible disease. If my MDs in Houston would have known what was going on with me in February with the onset of

original symptoms, I might not have disseminating VF. I would like to help educate the public about VF, and if it means taking legal action, "Count Me In."

Margaret P.
Tucson, Arizona
Contracted VF at age 38

I am currently under a doctor's care for my Valley Fever. My mother came out from California to help with the house and children for ten days at the height of my illness.

I changed doctors in the middle of my diagnosis. The first doctor didn't want to talk about Valley Fever. I brought up that I thought I might have it. He did not have a "plan of action" for whatever was causing my illness although all of my symptoms pointed to Valley Fever being the cause. The first blood test done by this doctor came back negative. The new doctor immediately said yes it is VF and re-ran the test which now came back positive.

K.C. H.
Heber City, Utah
Contracted VF at age 27 in Phoenix, Arizona

I had very good health prior to Valley Fever. I am newly diagnosed and have a new baby due in September. I don't know what the future will bring. I worked at a construction site in Phoenix, Arizona. I worked until I was so sick I couldn't take any more. We are seeing a pulmonary doctor in Provo, Utah. He doesn't know anything about this disease and researched it on the internet after I saw him. He is referring me to an ID specialist in Salt Lake.

There was a serious outbreak of Valley Fever in Utah. Prior to that outbreak it was not thought that Valley Fever spores could survive in cold weather areas. As a result of this outbreak, some Utah physicians are familiar with the disease. However, I am limited by my insurance as to whom I can see for the illness.

I am just hoping that someone can help me. I can't work anymore. My doctor is completing the paperwork for me to take medical leave from my work under the family leave act. I only get twelve weeks of leave.

I have been encouraged by several attorneys to apply immediately for SSI, but I have heard that it will be an uphill battle because of the lack of recognition of the disease and the severity with which its victims can be attacked.

I am living with my mother-in-law. My entire family is concerned because we have nothing to fall back on and no money to pay the bills. The future is a mystery right now.

I had to quit my job as a crane operator in Arizona and move back to Utah where my wife and kids were living so that my wife could take care of me. I was very sick and could not walk for more than five minutes at a time. I have had to claim bankruptcy because I could not work and had lots of bills to pay. There was no way to pay them. I wish I had known about the disease before working in Arizona.

Rudy V.
Bakersfield, California
Contracted VF at age 46

At present I am still fighting affects of Valley Fever. I no longer have control of my diabetes. I believe this is a direct result of contracting VF. I was diagnosed with a mild case of diabetes in 1994 and had it under control by 1996. I did not take medication until September 2001.

Seven weeks after contracting Valley Fever I lost control of my blood sugar. It shot up to 550 and affected my vision. I could not see clearly. That was an indicator that led to the discovery of my diabetes being out of control. My blood sugar will not go lower than 240. I just returned from Samsun Clinic in Santa Barbara and they are trying a new type of insulin on me. I miss the good health. It seems like I am a different person now.

Bill Kellogg (deceased)
Written by his sister, Lorrie.
Contracted VF at 22 years old
Orange, California

I stumbled onto your website completely by accident recently. I was going over further information regarding Valley Fever for a neighbor of mine who may or may not have the illness and I found your website very educational. I want to thank you for all the information about Valley Fever. My brother, Bill Kellogg, was only 22 when Valley Fever killed him on August 8, 1993. His death shocked, devastated and traumatized my entire family. Even after 11 years, my family has never been the same. This disease was completely unknown to us until we were told by the doctors that Bill had it. By the time they figured out what he had, it was too late and he died.

Bill had a hereditary kidney disease that left him in full kidney failure by 1992 and he was on dialysis for the last year of his life. Although he had kidney failure, he was still active as much as he could be. He worked part time as a physical education teacher for a Catholic elementary school in Orange, CA.

We believe he contracted the disease when he traveled through the San Joaquin Valley, California to visit a friend at UC Davis in April 1993. The symptoms remained dormant and it wasn't until days before my mom was due to donate a kidney to him in July 1993 that he became sick with Valley Fever.

He was sick for 3 weeks and the doctors thought he had pneumonia and were treating him for that. It wasn't until they realized he was getting worse, and that his breathing had become labored and he wasn't responding to the medications that treated pneumonia that they finally opened up his chest, looked inside, and sewed him back up and told us they were sorry but there was nothing they could do for us. Valley Fever had completely taken over his lungs and soon after the doctors had discovered that fact, my dear brother passed away.

None of my family had ever heard of the disease before we found out my brother had it. My brother had to pay the ultimate price for this illness. This horrible disease robbed him of life. It robbed him of his dream of having a family of his own. It robbed him of having his long time friends because they drifted away when he became so sick because they didn't know how to deal with it. It robbed my family of the sheer honor of his presence.

We all watched him suffer for days until he didn't want to even speak or eat. It was three weeks of hell watching him have to suffer and die that way! My brother was a wonderful person. He was so young and in the prime of his life. This should not have happened. My mom was days away from giving him a new life with a kidney to end his dialysis nightmare and live a healthy life. Unfortunately it was not to be.

Even after a decade, the healing hasn't mended the enormous hole that was left when Bill passed away. I wish you could have seen my family before Bill became sick. We were so close and a happy family. It all happened so quickly and what is really odd is that Bill was so scared of dying from the transplant operation! Little did any of us know it wouldn't be that at all but of something that none of us had ever heard about.

My brother was so amazing especially in the most difficult period of his life, the last year before he died. He was so strong and brave to endure dialysis three times a week and continue working at the school coaching sports for the kids. Where he found the energy only God knows! He was unable to accept a salary due to money he was receiving from the state to help pay for his expensive medical needs, so he worked for free and returned the salary money back into the sports program. That is just one example of the many reasons why he is remembered and honored each year at the annual sports banquet with an award and scholarship in his name for the top boy and girl athlete who have the desire, dedication, discipline and determination to be a top athlete. My family attends every year and are so proud that he has such a legacy.

I am impressed with the time and energy you have already spent on such an informative website. You told me things I didn't even know still about Valley Fever. I live in Santa Barbara County and can tell you that the other night on the news it was reported another 150 cases of Valley Fever in Ventura County alone have been documented. They believe the wild fires last fall in the area have caused this. It tore my heart to see a young lady (probably in her mid 20's) on tv crying about having Valley Fever and all she did was "breathe"...It was the first report I have ever seen on tv.

I am writing all this because I believe that misdiagnosis of Valley Fever is common and the lack of knowledge among doctors prevents many cases, like my brother's, to be treated properly. My brother is a part of this growing statistic that needs to be addressed. The doctors in Orange County, CA. were not familiar with the disease because they saw so few cases and did not catch on in time to have possibly saved my brother. His compromised immune system just added strikes to the situation and though they eventually diagnosed him correctly, he passed away within weeks of becoming ill.

My hope is that someday this disease gets the attention it deserves so that others can be saved before their lives are traumatically changed forever like ours is now. It is a little known illness with huge ramifications.

There is not enough information getting out to the public regarding this illness. I feel the areas that Valley Fever is prevalent such as California and Arizona have a moral responsibility to the public to address the risks and possibilities of contracting this disease. It is an ugly, horrible way to suffer and die. I know, I watched my brother for 3 weeks until it took him. He was way too young and had such a bright future. I hope I can help to make a difference.

The Future

Now that you have had the opportunity to read this book from cover to cover, you can understand why the need was there for a comprehensive book about this disease. Don't hesitate to refer to this book often. Many people have already told us they plan on purchasing a copy for their doctor, family, friends and co-workers.

Since 2002 we have been researching Valley Fever, talking with Valley Fever patients, and offering information and support via e-mail, phone and our web site, www.valleyfeversurvivor.com. Valley Fever Survivor will not stop working until there are national warnings about Valley Fever given to the traveling public, until residents of the endemic areas are told the truth about what it means to contract Valley Fever, and until there is a cure and vaccine for this presently incurable naturally occurring biohazard.

We are presently working on another book that will reveal every shocking detail about Valley Fever to the public. In that book *everything* the nation needs to know about the disease will finally be available. Included will be its history as a biological weapon as well as the distillation of over a hundred years of medical knowledge and the corresponding years of political inaction. It will also feature statistical analysis, further information on effects against specific races, more personal stories, the legal issues surrounding Valley Fever, how it affects homeland security, and much more.

The statistics from our web site's thousands of online form responses will be included, as will information about the financial, social, ethical, and legal consequences of the ongoing Valley Fever epidemic. It will also include expanded medical information from nearly a dozen interviews with the leading doctors and medical professionals on this disease.

The information about Valley Fever's effects on the military, local governments, and biological warfare is as gripping as any military thriller in the theaters. Many astonishing facts will be revealed for the first time ever in a book designed for the public at large. This book will also include hundreds of additional citations from peer reviewed medical journals, showing our readers the scientific support for our facts and findings.

Such an important, painstakingly researched book is not an easy task, considering the history of this disease. Decades of secrets about this disease have been buried by the misconception that Valley Fever is not a big deal, but the truth is plain to see for anyone who does thorough research. While these little known facts are fascinating and deserve to be publicized for the sake of public health, nothing is more important than helping people learn the truth about this disease and promoting the vaccine and cure.

Since there are some things people need to know *now*, we knew *Valley Fever Epidemic* must be released first. Please tell others about this book. The information here could help save lives.

Valley Fever Survivor leads the charge in patient support with our message board, which serves as the hub of the worldwide Valley Fever community. In 2007, VFS along with our Phoenix/Glendale Valley Fever Survivor Support Group held the first Valley Fever Survivor Benefit for a Vaccine and Cure. It featured Dr. Garry Cole, a world leading Valley Fever vaccine researcher.

We worked to notify our readers about Valley Fever related political issues so everyone would know to contact their legislative representatives on issues like nikkomycin Z and vaccine funding. Our 2006 petition had thousands of signatures from people in dozens of states to assist California Representative William Thomas achieve federal backing for California's Valley Fever Vaccine Project, which was successfully accepted into the Tax Relief and Health Care Act of 2006. With our supporters, we continue in the fight to appropriate money for this cause with Representative Thomas' successor Representative Kevin McCarthy.

Beyond issues of research funding, Valley Fever Survivor has continued efforts for patient support, provided technical documentation to assist veterans to successfully receive compensation when their Valley Fever has a service connection, assisted others in their legal proceedings, and more.

None of our accomplishments were done with a paid staff of coordinated media professionals. All of our work was completed by volunteers: Authors David and Sharon, Valley Fever Survivor Support Group Directors and their families, VFS Support Group members, and www.valleyfeversurvivor.com readers who recognized the importance of this disease, read about the ways they could participate, and decided they wanted to make a difference.

The Need for Action

Valley Fever Survivor coined the term SARFI in 2003. SARFI stands for Serious Acute Respiratory Fungal Infection as another way of describing coccidioidomycosis (Valley Fever). We had hoped that by using the term "SARFI," the CDC could find parallels with the highly publicized, similar sounding disease SARS.

After all, SARS was important enough for national and international media attention and the CDC made sure to warn travelers with information about SARS. By contrast, the Valley Fever epidemic affects far more people and is deserving of warnings on TV, radio, and other media. Unfortunately, such warnings have not occurred to date. There should have been a tidal wave of national news media attention on Valley Fever years ago, just as there should be today, but instead it has been kept a "local secret."[100]

Please visit our web site's letters page http://www.valleyfeversurvivor.com/letters.html to read our CDC action letters and perhaps you will write a letter of your own.

SARFI will be an important figure in the fight to get warnings out about Valley Fever. You can look for our SARFI mascot in future educational materials and projects.

SARS, Mad Cow, West Nile, Tuberculosis and other diseases are obviously important but so is SARFI. Don't forget, this is not just a fungal infection but the disease is caused by the most virulent fungal parasite known to man and is the only fungus regulated by two antiterrorism laws. Once the spore is inhaled, this dimorphic fungus becomes a parasite in its host. You should remember that there is no cure for Valley Fever and the disease can be lethal even decades later. Furthermore, with the continuing increase in population in the hyperendemic areas, the epidemic is expected to continue.

According to the Valley Fever Center for Excellence's 2003 Annual Report, "the State of Arizona has not perceived nor dealt with Valley Fever as an emerging health problem which could threaten future population growth, commerce, and tourism. This attitude and perception:

- leads to a non-committal approach to the awareness of Valley Fever as an emerging infectious disease issue.
- raise[s] doubts about the willingness of the State of Arizona to "take responsibility" for its endemic disease and care for the public health of its citizens and visitors.
- compromises public relations and economic development opportunities.
- complicates requesting support for state and local funding for Valley Fever education and research.
- tends to keep Valley Fever a "local secret" because of fears of scaring off individuals and commercial interests which might be interested in locating to this area.

"The University of Arizona and the State of Arizona need to re-evaluate their perception and attitudes toward Valley Fever, accept ownership of this disease and provide the VFCE necessary resources for the support of its core programs."[100]

The VFCE's Dr. John Galgiani was featured in a KVOA news story on September 24, 2004.[205] He told KVOA that "Valley Fever poses a bioterrorist threat, perhaps even more dangerous than anthrax," and that the number of people diagnosed with Valley Fever infections in 2004 was "more than any other year this reportable disease has been tracked in the state of Arizona." The caseload was considerably higher in every subsequent year.

Thousands are diagnosed with Valley Fever every year and hundreds of thousands more are unknowingly infected, but it is important to look beyond the statistics; the toll it takes on each individual is incalculable. Beverly Lobenstein, one of our Support Group Directors, wrote the following when lung surgery was proposed for her case:

My condition has worsened to the point where they are going to remove my left lung. For the last 9 weeks I have had to be on Amphotericin B IV's everyday. I am inoperable at this time due to the infection being so bad. I am told I will die with this...That the surgery will only buy me a little more time.

I will never see my grandsons grow up. I will never see them graduate or marry. I will never live a full life as I once did, never do all the fun things I used to do. Rather I must be happy with what is left of my life...make the best of what time I do have, forget all my hopes and dreams...just live each day as it comes.

I still cry about this. I still hurt in my heart over this. I am sorry for all those who become like me, and those who are way worse then me. I know I too at some point will be one of those way worse people and that is what I have to look forward to. I would not wish this upon anyone.

The people of Arizona and the nation have the right to know what is in their soil and air, how dangerous it is to their health, and that there is something they can do about it. Everyone needs to speak up. Each and every voice the politicians hear can only lead to positive change. Together we can eradicate this disease once and for all, but we need your help.

Our Work Continues

Because people should have the right to decide what kind of health risks they are willing to endure, Valley Fever needs publicity and warnings for potential visitors and residents. The disease also needs a vaccine to protect the millions of people who visit, pass through, and live in the endemic areas. Finally, this incurable disease needs a cure so the residents of, the veterans stationed in and passing through, and the tourists to these areas who are already infected will never need to fear a Valley Fever reactivation or reinfection.

We will not stop working toward these goals until this devastating disease has been defeated.

To contact the authors, David and Sharon, please write to voiceforaction@valleyfeversurvivor.com

Everyone is encouraged to visit our web site, www.valleyfeversurvivor.com and participate in our online surveys to be included in the statistical analysis in our major upcoming book on coccidioidomycosis.

Appendix A: Organizations and Internet Resources

There is a great deal of work ahead in the fight against coccidioidomycosis. Although there are already organizations dedicated to fighting Valley Fever, and even chances at state and federal funding, none have even come close to the amount of support they need. Please consider donating to or volunteering with some of these organizations.

Valley Fever Advocacy and Research Organizations

Valley Fever Survivor

http://www.valleyfeversurvivor.com

Valley Fever Survivor is the only Internet site completely dedicated to advocacy and to the release of up-to-date and accurate information about Valley Fever based on peer reviewed medical research. Readers can also review our previous and ongoing political actions and read the political letters we had sent.

The Valley Fever Survivor Message Board has become the hub of the Internet Valley Fever community, with thousands of posts from hundreds of members. The Valley Fever Survivor Support Groups have organized meetings to provide comfort to those infected with Valley Fever and are planning fundraising and publicity programs as well.

Hats, T-shirts, mugs and other items can be purchased from the Valley Fever Survivor online store.

Profits from the sale of these items will be used to cover our expenses, promotion, lobbying, and our other efforts to educate and promote awareness of Valley Fever. Please visit our online store to learn more:

http://www.valleyfeversurvivor.com/store.html

The University of Texas San Antonio Valley Fever Vaccine Project.

We urge everyone to donate generously to support this important research. Dr. Garry Cole at UTSA is working on a new vaccine that may not only protect people from Valley Fever, but may even work as a cure in patients with Valley Fever. Early testing has shown it to be 100% effective in mice, but more advanced testing is needed to determine its true effectiveness.

In his decades of work Dr. Cole has published nearly 200 peer reviewed medical articles and held positions with the International Union of Microbiological Societies, the National Institutes of Health, and many other medical organizations. Recently he was a Stranahan Endowed Research Chair at the Department of Microbiology and Immunology at the Medical University of Ohio until becoming a Professor and the Margaret Batts Tobin Endowed Chair at the UTSA in the Department of Biology. His faculty homepage is:
http://bio.utsa.edu/faculty/cole.html

Donations by check should indicate that it is for "Valley Fever vaccine research" in the memo area of the check or in an accompanying letter or note. Checks should be payable to UTSA and mailed to the following address:

Dr. Garry Cole
The University of Texas at San Antonio
One UTSA Circle
Room MBT 1.308
San Antonio, TX 78249

Credit card donations are also possible with MasterCard, Visa, American Express and Discover. These contributions can be made online through the Development Office's giving site:
https://secure.entango.com/donate/Up3sjqiUrnB

UTSA has informed us that this is a secure web site and that an acknowledgment letter will be sent to every donor. The letter can be used as a receipt for tax purposes. Although the University's tax ID is not necessary, donors who wish to have the tax ID may contact the UTSA Development Office at 210-458-4130. Along with your donation, please let them know you heard about Dr. Cole's research from Valley Fever Survivor.

Rotary District 5240's Valley Fever Vaccine Project of the Americas

www.valleyfever.com

This is the homepage to the Valley Fever Americas Foundation Rotary District 5240 project dedicated to raising funds to help support the vaccine research being coordinated through the Valley Fever Vaccine Project. As the name suggests, their primary purpose is to develop a vaccine to prevent future infections from this disease. Their work is of the utmost importance and requires your support. The web site offers a seasonal newsletter to keep readers updated on the status of vaccine research and funding.

To donate, please send your checks to:

Valley Fever Americas Foundation
PO Box 2752
Bakersfield, California 93303
Tax ID # 77-0424552

As noted on their web site, contributions to the Valley Fever Vaccine Project are not only tax deductible but "100 percent of all corporate and individual contributions will be allocated to the research, development or clinical testing costs in the development of a vaccine for Valley Fever. Overhead is completely provided by fundraising and contributions from Rotary Clubs and by contributions by the project predecessor, Valley Fever Research Foundation."

The Valley Fever Center for Excellence

The Valley Fever Center for Excellence (VFCE) is associated with the University of Arizona and presently conducting medical research for better medication and treatment for those with Valley Fever. The University of Arizona is conducting experiments with nikkomycin Z, an experimental drug that has been suspected for decades to be a cure for Valley Fever. In September 2007, the VFCE announced that it successfully acquired a one million dollar FDA grant for

nikkomycin Z research. Contributions for this research can be
sent to the following address:

The University of Arizona
Valley Fever Center for Excellence
Mail Stop 1-111INF
3601 S. 6th Avenue
Tucson, Arizona 85723

Please make the check out to the University of Arizona
Foundation. You need to stipulate on your check's memo line
that this donation is for nikkomycin Z research only and include
the tax ID number below. Along with your check be sure to
include a letter or note with the following information:

1. State that your contribution is only for the nikkomycin Z
    research project.
2. This contribution is to go to the VFCE tax ID number 86-
    6004791.
3. State that you received this information from Valley Fever
    Survivor.
4. Request a receipt for your donation.

Other Groups of Interest

The Partnership for Prescription Assistance (PPA)
http://www.pparx.org

The PPA is an alliance of pharmaceutical companies that
helps patients to receive drugs they might not otherwise be able
to afford. Information about this service can be read at the link
above (be sure cookies are enabled in your web browser). The
PPA can also be reached through their telephone number 1-888-
4PPA-NOW (1-888-477-2669).

The Pfizer Philanthropy Program

http://www.pfizer.com/pfizer/subsites/philanthropy/access/index.jsp

The pharmaceutical company Pfizer Inc. may be able to assist you with the high cost of Valley Fever treatments. See if you qualify for any of their programs at the link above or visit their main page www.pfizer.com for more information. You should also ask your doctor whether your current medication's manufacturer has a similar program.

IMOM

www.imom.org

Since Valley Fever affects so many animals it is important to mention the charitable organization IMOM. Their web site's front page states that they "are dedicated to insure that no companion animal has to be euthanized simply because their caretaker is financially challenged." The costs of Valley Fever's treatment can be so high that organizations like imom.org may be essential for many pet owners living in endemic areas.

The Fungal Research Trust

http://fungalresearchtrust.org

This site has useful information about fungi and antifungal drugs. Valley Fever sufferers should be particularly interested in the list of side effects.

Appendix B: Essential Facts

Through my years of research into medical journals, medical conference transcripts, interviews, and surveys and questionnaires from those suffering from Valley Fever, I have seen the horrors this disease can create.

The morbidity from Valley Fever is worse than the mortality because many people lose more than their health. The fatigue, pain, surgeries and debilitation have resulted in high medical expenses and caused the type of strain that forces people to lose their jobs, spouses, families, insurance, and sometimes their homes. Many patients with Valley Fever have fallen between the cracks for years because the medical community is often unaware of the seriousness of this disease or is working with outdated and misleading information.

Only by researching Valley Fever's medical and military history and using the most up-to-date information can anyone truly understand the danger posed by this disease. When all the research data is considered, Valley Fever is clearly not rare, not benign, and is an ongoing national catastrophe of epidemic proportions.

The following list of annotated Valley Fever facts attests to this. To add to the usefulness of this book, a vast array of Valley Fever facts were condensed to only a few pages. Any novice can now get up to speed with the most important information quickly, and anyone considering a trip to an endemic area can quickly see and judge the consequences of such a decision.

Since earlier versions of these facts had previously been used in legal proceedings, this appendix's bibliography has not been integrated with the rest of this book's bibliographical notes. This way you may copy these pages and their corresponding citations for more convenient use in your own legal proceedings, if necessary.

Fungi of the genus *Coccidioides* cause the disease coccidioidomycosis, more commonly known as Valley Fever.

In the United States, *Coccidioides* spp. can grow in Arizona, California, New Mexico, Nevada, Texas and Utah so the fungus is considered *endemic* to these areas and Valley Fever is an endemic disease there. It is estimated that 65% of Valley Fever cases in the United States are contracted in Arizona and that a third are contracted in California. There is virtually no tracking in other endemic areas.

There is no cure for Valley Fever. Treatment often fails, leading to relapses in up to 50% of cases, and misdiagnoses are common (1-3). Incorrect medical treatment, as with corticosteroids, can exacerbate the disease (4). Patients may require expensive lifelong treatment when the disease becomes severe (medication can be $20,000 per year) and it may cost two-thirds of a million dollars for lifetime treatment (5, 6).

Doctors are frequently not educated about the seriousness of Valley Fever. This prompted the State of Arizona in 2006 to spend $50,000 to provide basic Valley Fever education for medical professionals.

While older data suggests symptoms occur in 40% of infections, recent data shows the disease seems to cause symptoms more frequently. Over half of those with Valley Fever suffer symptoms initially and many will have their infections reactivate later. In some cases the disease waxes and wanes or remains chronic to create a lifetime of suffering (29). To date, no research is available to know how many of the initially asymptomatic cases are likely to activate.

Coccidioides is a dimorphic fungus, meaning it changes from its soil-dwelling form into a parasite when it is inhaled. *Coccidioides* spores are easily inhaled, roughly the same size as anthrax spores, classified as naturally occurring biohazards, and the most virulent fungus known to man (7). Only one spore is needed to be inhaled for a lifelong infection (8). These spores are dangerous enough that anyone culturing them is required to use a Biosafety Level III laboratory. This requirement is only one step below the measures of safety needed to handle Ebola, the infamously dangerous hemorrhagic fever virus.

To indicate the level of danger posed by *Coccidioides*, it is regulated by the federal government as a Select Agent in the Antiterrorism and Effective Death Penalty Act of 1996 and the Public Health Security and Bioterrorism Preparedness and Response Act of 2002. The CDC reserves the Select Agent list for toxins and biological agents "that have the potential to pose a severe threat to public health and safety." *Coccidioides* is the only genus of fungi presently on that list (9).

Dr. John Galgiani of the Valley Fever Center for Excellence (VFCE) stated to the Arizona State Legislature's Committee on Health that the Valley Fever epidemic could be the result of a terrorist attack. At this same meeting, he also observed that increased construction in Arizona might also lead to increased infection rates (6).

During World War II, some captured Nazi prisoners of war were held in Florence, Arizona. Many of these prisoners subsequently fell ill after being infected by Valley Fever. Although Nazi concentration camps were infamous for their torture and cruelty, Germany invoked the Geneva Convention because they felt it was a violation of prisoner's rights for America to keep prisoners of war in areas where Valley Fever could be contracted. America obliged them on this request, although American soldiers are still stationed in endemic areas and American civilians can freely visit or live in areas with the disease that was considered too cruel for Nazi prisoners (10-13).

Since it was estimated that 3% of the population in the USA's endemic counties are infected annually (14), year 2000 census estimates show that approximately 200,000 residents were infected with this disease each year. In five years this means 1,000,000 people will have been infected with this incurable disease. Many people may have this in their bodies and not know it yet. It is like a ticking time bomb waiting to go off. The population and diagnoses of infections have increased so quickly that it may take even less than three years for a million new Valley Fever infections to occur.

Another estimate of the overall Valley Fever infection rate is that approximately only 2% of infections are clinically diagnosed (57). In Arizona the number of reported Valley Fever case diagnoses was 5,535 for 2006. If these diagnoses were only two percent, then over 276,000 people are estimated to have been infected in Arizona in 2006. The 5,535 cases reported from Arizona is a 46% increase over the previous year's 3,778 reported cases. California has reported 3,131 cases of Valley Fever for 2006. The CDC's total number of nationally reported Valley Fever cases in 2006 is 8,916. The national number of infections for 2006 is therefore estimated to be over 445,000 new infections. 2006 far exceeded any previous year as history's worst epidemic of this incurable disease by a wide margin, and provisional infection reporting from 2007 was nearly as bad.

"Cases are notoriously underreported" (15) and the actual number of infected persons may be even higher since countless visitors are infected as well. They often return to their home states and countries where the disease is less well known and less likely to be diagnosed correctly (7, 16, 17).

A 2006 study showed that 29% of community-acquired pneumonia cases in Arizona were caused by Valley Fever. Doctors believe 29% is an "underestimate" of the actual cases of Valley Fever pneumonia due to factors involved in the study (56).

A brief mention of the ongoing Valley Fever epidemic finally appeared on Arizona's Department of Health Services web site next to a warning about the 2006 E. coli spinach scare, and later as a separate web page in 2007, but there is no policy to warn potential visitors of the danger. Serious Valley Fever infections have been reported in people who had simply driven through (18-21) or had flown on a plane that had passed through endemic areas (22).

Occupational Valley Fever lawsuits have often been successful. One example is of a man infected with Valley Fever in the course of his job as a trucker. He was successfully able to litigate his case to force his employers to pay monetary damages for having him travel into harm's way in Pressley v. Southwestern Freight Lines and Liberty Mutual Insurance Co. 114 N.C. App. 342, 551 W.E. 2d 118.

Dust control is essential with Valley Fever because "soil disturbance[s] (with the subsequent formation of dust) and extensive outdoor activity enhance the chances of infection" (24) and when dust control does not occur at places like construction sites and places with exposed soil, it creates an enhanced Valley Fever risk for employees and everyone nearby (20, 25, 26).

For decades, it has been known that Valley Fever can spread to attack any organ of the body (18). This is called dissemination. On the skin, disseminated Valley Fever can cause disfigurement (30), in the spine it can cause paralysis, (31, 32) in bones it may calcify or create necrotic, rotting, liquefying lesions that require amputation of limbs (33-35), and it can kill patients when striking at and near critical organs like the lungs, heart and brain (36-38). It can also induce mental state changes in its victims (39) including memory loss (40).

In the United States, the medical treatment of Valley Fever each year creates "an estimated total cost of 120 million dollars. Unfortunately, the rates of failure and relapse after treatment of chronic pulmonary or disseminated Coccidioidomycosis are disappointingly high." (27)

There is no way to ensure that a patient will not have a reactivation or to predict how Valley Fever will manifest itself. A severe reactivation of Valley Fever can occur decades after the first infection and in unexpected ways. This was demonstrated in the case of a man who worked briefly in a Valley Fever endemic area. When he was infected in 1957 he experienced pneumonia and appeared to recover. In 1958 he had a reactivation of his

Valley Fever that required the removal of a testicle and other parts of his genitourinary tract. Again the Valley Fever went dormant, until it reactivated over four decades later as meningitis in 2002 to kill him. Even when an infected person does not look or feel sick, reactivation is always a dangerous lingering possibility with this disease (28).

Valley Fever can cause arthritis, synovitis and other maladies that cause joint pains, myalgias (muscle pains), and severe fatigue. Since the disease is often undiagnosed or misdiagnosed, it may be responsible for millions of Chronic Fatigue Syndrome and Fibromyalgia diagnoses. It may also account for a large percentage of America's 70 million people with arthritis or chronic joint pain.

Recent Valley Fever studies have shown an 8.5% death rate in children (58), a 53% death rate in those with pericardial symptoms (42) and a 26.8% death rate in senior citizens with the disease (43).

Since animals can also be infected with the disease, even our pets are not safe. One study of previously healthy dogs in Arizona showed that 27% became infected with Valley Fever within two years (44). Over $6 million of veterinary expenses for Valley Fever are estimated annually in Pima County alone (45).

Although anyone can suffer a severe or fatal case of this disease, Valley Fever is often more serious in Asians, African Americans, Hispanics, and Native Americans (5, 37, 46-48). Filipinos had death rates as high as 192 times those of Caucasians and African Americans died of Valley Fever up to 23 times more frequently than Caucasians. This is undoubtedly why *Coccidioides* spores were considered as a race-specific biological weapon and held in Fort Detrick by the CIA during the Cold War (49).

Overall, more healthy people are infected with Valley Fever than immunocompromised people and no deficiencies are necessary to get a severe or fatal case (19, 50). Only 12% of hospitalized Valley Fever patients in a recent national study had any immune system compromising conditions whatsoever (58). Immune deficiencies from organ transplantation, diabetes, HIV/AIDS, certain medications, and other conditions, however, can allow the disease to take hold faster and with more severity than it might otherwise (16). Even physical injuries and seemingly ordinary surgeries can prompt the reactivation of a latent infection (51, 52). A "health safety net" of sorts vanishes once a person has Valley Fever because many factors can increase the risk of reactivation.

Misleading and outdated medical information has unfortunately been repeated for far too long. It has led to many misconceptions among doctors who do not have time for an in-depth study of the medical literature. Among the misconceptions are statements that Valley Fever cannot reactivate (it has in many patients, even those treated with medicine), that symptoms will not last longer than one year (as it has become chronic in many patients), and that a patient must be of a specific race or have an immune problem for a case to become serious (which ignores the fact that anyone can die or suffer from the disease).

As to why local residents don't seem to take the disease seriously, "...too often Valley Fever is still perceived as simply an annoyance by the general public, health care professionals and local government officials. Even the majority of local residents in the endemic area perceive Valley Fever as a relatively benign disease. Combining this misperception with the lack of knowledge about the disease among new residents, tourists, new businesses, athletes and students moving into the endemic area, creates a vast population base which must endure Valley Fever illnesses (often without an accurate diagnosis) while being unprepared to deal with any possible complications arising from a *Coccidioides* sp. infection." (53)

"In Arizona, California, and Texas, increasing numbers of residents are affected by coccidioidomycosis. As a result, employers in these areas increasingly face lost days from work and substantial medical costs attributable to coccidioidal disease. Such organizations as the military, schools, travel agencies, and employers with national applicant pools actually create the opportunity for groups to relocate to or visit endemic regions, with subsequent risk for exposure...it is almost certain that some persons will become seriously ill." (16)

"Care for coccidioidomycosis will continue to drain health care resources as long as the epidemic continues. Indirect costs are also important as patients are removed from the workforce. Commerce in the Central Valley [of California] may have also suffered as businesses may be reluctant to locate there, conventions stay away, and tourists revise travel plans. Clearly, the economic costs of coccidioidomycosis extend well beyond patient care." (26)

"Coccidioidomycosis has long been recognized as one of the most difficult endemic mycoses to treat." (2)

"The inhalation of the highly infectious arthrospores of *Coccidioides immitis* can produce a host response ranging from a simple flulike syndrome to widespread dissemination, possibly involving every organ of the body and not infrequently ending fatally." (54)

"The cost of antifungal medication is high, in the range of $5000-$20,000 per year of treatment. For managing critically ill patients with coccidioidomycosis, there are considerable additional costs including intensive care support for many days or weeks." (3)

"The rapid and increasing influx of industry and agriculture into the southwestern United States has heightened the importance of coccidioidomycosis as an occupational disease. Before 1938, this disease was of little interest because relatively few clinical cases were recognized and the morbidity caused by primary infection was not appreciated...the introduction of industrial or agricultural workers into endemic areas carries with it the responsibility of assessing the hazard of the disease to such population." (25) Naturally, the moral responsibility also extends to people affected by such work, some of whom may simply be passing through town but will have a lifelong infection.

"...the State of Arizona has not perceived nor dealt with Valley Fever as an emerging health problem which could threaten future population growth, commerce, and tourism. This attitude and perception:

- leads to a non-committal approach to the awareness of Valley Fever as an emerging infectious disease issue.
- raise[s] doubts about the willingness of the State of Arizona to 'take responsibility' for its endemic disease and care for the public health of its citizens and visitors.
- compromises public relations and economic development opportunities.
- complicates requesting support for state and local funding for Valley Fever education and research.
- tends to keep Valley Fever a 'local secret' because of fears of scaring off individuals and commercial interests which might be interested in locating to this area.

"The University of Arizona and the State of Arizona need to re-evaluate their perception and attitudes toward Valley Fever, accept ownership of this disease and provide the VFCE [the organization making this statement] necessary resources for the support of its core programs." (55)

"Since Valley Fever is an inherent problem of the Southwest, it is a regional disease (with national and international implications) that the people of the Southwest must recognize and accept as their responsibility...So in answer to the question, 'Who is responsible?' Very simply, [as residents of the Southwest] 'We are!'" (53)

Essential Facts Endnotes

1. Graybill JR. Future directions of antifungal chemotherapy. Clin Infect Dis. 1992 Mar;14 Suppl 1:S170-81.

2. Oldfield EC 3rd, Bone WD, Martin CR, Gray GC, Olson P, Schillaci RF. Prediction of relapse after treatment of coccidioidomycosis. Clin Infect Dis. 1997 Nov;25(5):1205-10.

3. Galgiani JN, Ampel NM, Catanzaro A, Johnson RH, Stevens DA, Williams PL. Practice guideline for the treatment of coccidioidomycosis. Infectious Diseases Society of America. Clin Infect Dis. 2000 Apr;30(4):658-61. Epub 2000 Apr 20.

4. DiCaudo DJ, Ortiz KJ, Mengden SJ, Lim KK. Sweet syndrome (acute febrile neutrophilic dermatosis) associated with pulmonary coccidioidomycosis. Arch Dermatol. 2005 Jul;141(7):881-4.

5. Chiller TM, Galgiani JN, Stevens DA. Coccidioidomycosis. Infect Dis Clin North Am. 2003 Mar;17(1):41-57, viii.

6. Arizona State Senate. 46th Legislature, First Regular Session. Minutes of Committee on Health. February 13, 2003. http://www.azleg.state.az.us/FormatDocument.asp?inDoc=/legtext/46leg/1R/comm_min/Senate/0213+HEA%2EDOC.htm Accessed March 29, 2004.

7. Dixon DM. Coccidioides immitis as a Select Agent of bioterrorism. J Appl Microbiol. 2001 Oct;91(4):602-5.

8. Copeland B, White D, Buenting J. Coccidioidomycosis of the head and neck. Ann Otol Rhinol Laryngol 2003 Jan;112(1):98-101.

9. CDC Select Agent Program Homepage. http://www.cdc.gov/od/sap/ Accessed 09/07/05.

10. Drutz DJ, Catanzaro A: Coccidioidomycosis. Part I. Am Rev Respir Dis 1978 Mar; 117(3): 559-85.

11. Deresinski SC. History of coccidioidomycosis: Dust to Dust. in Stevens DA, ed. Coccidioidomycosis. A Text. New York, London: Plenum Medical Book Company, 1980: p1-20.

12. Hugenholtz PG. Climate and coccidioidomycosis. In Ferguson MS, ed. Proceedings of Symposium on Coccidioidomycosis. Atlanta, Public Health Service Publication No. 575, 1957: p136-143.

13. Smith CE. Reminisces of the Flying Chlamydospore and its allies. In Ajello L, ed. Coccidioidomycosis. Papers from the second symposium on coccidioidomycosis. Tucson: University of Arizona Press, 1967: xiii-xxii.

14. VFCE, personal communication.

15. Howard DH. The epidemiology and ecology of blastomycosis, coccidioidomycosis and histoplasmosis. Zentralbl Bakteriol Mikrobiol Hyg [A]. 1984 Jul;257(2):219-27.

16. Galgiani JN. Coccidioidomycosis: a regional disease of national importance. Rethinking approaches for control. Ann Intern Med. 1999 Feb 16;130(4 Pt 1):293-300.

17. Standaert SM, Schaffner W, Galgiani JN, Pinner RW, Kaufman L, Durry E, Hutcheson RH. Coccidioidomycosis among visitors to a Coccidioides immitis-endemic area: an outbreak in a military reserve unit. J Infect Dis 1995 Jun;171(6):1672-5.

18. Fiese MJ. Coccidioidomycosis. Springfield, Charles C. Thomas, 1958.

19. Bouza E, Dreyer JS, Hewitt WL, Meyer RD. Coccidioidal meningitis. An analysis of thirty-one cases and review of the literature. Medicine (Baltimore) 1981 May;60(3):139-72.

20. Kirkland TN, Fierer J. Coccidioidomycosis: a reemerging infectious disease. Emerg Infect Dis. 1996 Jul-Sep;2(3):192-9.

21. Wu J, Linscott AJ, Oberle A, Fowler M. Pathology case of the month. Occupational hazard? Coccidioidomycosis (Coccidioides immitis). J La State Med Soc. 2003 Jul-Aug;155(4):187-8.

22. Papadopoulos KI, Castor B, Klingspor L, Dejmek A, Loren I, Bramnert M. Bilateral isolated adrenal coccidioidomycosis. J Intern Med. 1996 Mar;239(3):275-8.

23. DiSalvo A. Dimorphic Fungi. Microbiology and Immunology On-Line. http://www.med.sc.edu:85/mycology/mycology-6.htm Accessed 13 July 2004.

24. Saubolle MA. Life Cycle and epidemiology of Coccidioides immitis. In: Einstein HE, Catanzaro A, eds. Coccidioidomycosis. Proceedings of the 5th International Conference on Coccidioidomycosis. Stanford University, 24-27 August, 1994. Washington, DC. National Foundation for Infectious Diseases; 1996: 1-8.

25. Schmelzer L, Tabershaw IB. Exposure factors in occupational coccidioidomycosis. Am J Public Health. 1968; 58:107-113.

26. Werner SB, Vugia DJ, Duffey P, Williamson J, Bissell S, Jackson RJ, Rutherford GW. California Department of Health Services' Policy Statement on Coccidioidomycosis. In: Einstein HE, Catanzaro A, eds. Coccidioidomycosis. Proceedings of the 5th International Conference on Coccidioidomycosis. Stanford University, 24-27 August, 1994. Washington, DC. National Foundation for Infectious Diseases; 1996: 363-372.

27. Laniado-Laborín R. Cost-benefit analysis of treating acute coccidioidal pneumonia with azole drugs. In: Proceedings of the Forty-Fifth Annual Coccidioidomycosis Study Group Meeting. March 31, 2001. The University of Arizona. Tucson, Arizona. http://www.vfce.arizona.edu/csg/csg45.htm Accessed 6/13/05.

28. Johnson R, Einstein H. Forty-five years of disseminated coccidioidomycosis. In: Proceedings of the Forty-Sixth Annual Coccidioidomycosis Study Group Meeting. March 31, 2001. The University of Arizona. April 6, 2002. Davis, California. VFCE. http://www.vfce.arizona.edu/csg/csg45.htm Accessed 6/13/05.

29. Cole GT, Xue JM, Okeke CN, Tarcha EJ, Basrur V, Schaller RA, Herr RA, Yu JJ, Hung CY. A vaccine against coccidioidomycosis is justified and attainable. Med Mycol. 2004 Jun;42(3):189-216.

30. Rance BR, Elston DM. Disseminated coccidioidomycosis discovered during routine skin cancer screening. Cutis 2002 Jul;70(1):70-2.

31. Iger M. Coccidioidal osteomyelitis. In: Ajello L, ed. Coccidioidomycosis: Current clinical and diagnostic status. Miami: Symposia Specialists; 1977: 177-190.

32. Pappagianis D. Clinical presentation of Infectious Entities. In: Einstein HE, Catanzaro A, eds. Coccidioidomycosis. Proceedings of the 5th International Conference on Coccidioidomycosis. Stanford University, 24-27 August, 1994. Washington, DC. National Foundation for Infectious Diseases; 1996: 9-11.

33. Rothman PE, Graw RG Jr, Harris JC Jr, Onslow JM. Coccidiodomycosis--possible fomite transmission. A review and report of a case. Am J Dis Child. 1969 Nov;118(5):792-801.

34. Deresinski SC. Coccidioidomycosis of bone and joints. In: Stevens DA. Coccidioidomycosis. A Text. New York, London: Plenum Medical Book Company, 1980: 195-211.

35. Winter WG Jr, Larson RK, Honeggar MM, Jacobsen DT, Pappagianis D, Huntington RW Jr. Coccidioidal arthritis and its treatment. J Bone Joint Surg Am. 1975; 57:1152-1157. Cited in: Holley K, Muldoon M, Tasker S. Coccidioides immitis osteomyelitis: a case series review. Orthopedics 2002 Aug;25(8):827-31, 831-2.

36. Catanzaro A, Drutz DJ. Pulmonary Coccidioidomycosis. In: Stevens DA. Coccidioidomycosis. A Text. New York, London: Plenum Medical Book Company, 1980: 147-161.

37. Einstein HE, Johnson RH. Coccidioidomycosis: new aspects of epidemiology and therapy. Clin Infect Dis 1993;16:349-56.

38. Reuss CS, Hall MC, Blair JE, Yeo T, Leslie KO. Endocarditis caused by Coccidioides species. Mayo Clin Proc. 2004 Nov;79(11):1451-4.

39. Hsue G, Napier JT, Prince RA, Chi J, Hospenthal DR. Treatment of meningeal coccidioidomycosis with caspofungin. J Antimicrob Chemother. 2004 Jul;54(1):292-4. Epub 2004 Jun 09.

40. Snyder CH. Coccidioidal meningitis presenting as memory loss. J Am Acad Nurse Pract. 2005 May;17(5):181-6.

41. Chu JH, Zaoutis TE, Argon J, Feudtner C. National epidemiology of endemic fungal infections in children. Public Health and the Environment. The 132nd Annual Meeting (November 6-10, 2004) of the American Public Health Association (APHA). http://apha.confex.com/apha/132am/techprogram/paper_89147.htm Accessed 2006 Aug 2.

42. Arsura EL, Bobba RK, Reddy CM. Coccidioidal pericarditis: a case presentation and review of the literature. Int J Infect Dis. 2005 Mar;9(2):104-9.

43. Arsura EL. The association of age and mortality in coccidioidomycosis [letter]. J Am Geriatr Soc 1997;45:532-3.

44. Shubitz LE, Butkiewicz CD, Dial SM, Lindan CP. Incidence of coccidioides infection among dogs residing in a region in which the organism is endemic. J Am Vet Med Assoc. 2005 Jun 1;226(11):1846-50.

45. Larson S, (ed). Canine study nears completion. Valley Fever Vaccine Project of the Americas Quarterly Newsletter. Vol: 6, No: 4. Bakersfield, CA. DB & Co., 2003.

46. Merck. Coccidioidomycosis. The Merck Manual of Diagnosis and Therapy. Sec. 13, Ch. 158, Systemic Fungal Diseases. http://www.merck.com/mrkshared/mmanual/section13/chapter158/158c.jsp Accessed 14 July 2004.

47. Rosenstein NE, Emery KW, Werner SB, Kao A, Johnson R, Rogers D, Vugia D, Reingold A, Talbot R, Plikaytis BD, Perkins BA, Hajjeh RA. Risk factors for severe pulmonary and disseminated coccidioidomycosis: Kern County, California, 1995-1996. Clin Infect Dis. 2001 Mar 1;32(5):708-15. Epub 2001 Feb 28.

48. Smith CE, Beard RR, Whiting EG, Rosenberg HG. Varieties of coccidioidal infection in relation to the epidemiology and control of diseases. Am J Public Health 1946;36:1394-1402.

49. Miller J, Engelberg S, Broad WJ. Germs: biological weapons and America's secret war. New York: Simon & Schuster, 2001.

50. Crum NF, Lederman ER, Hale BR, Lim ML, Wallace MR. A cluster of disseminated coccidioidomycosis cases at a US military hospital. Mil Med. 2003 Jun;168(6):460-4.

51. Pappagianis D. The phenomenon of locus minoris resistentiae in coccidioidomycosis. In: Einstein HE, Catanzaro A, eds. Coccidioidomycosis. Proceedings of the 4th International Conference on Coccidioidomycosis. Washington, DC. National Foundation for Infectious Diseases; 1985: 319-329.

52. Caraway NP, Fanning CV, Stewart JM, Tarrand JJ, Weber KL. Coccidioidomycosis osteomyelitis masquerading as a bone tumor. A report of 2 cases. Acta Cytol. 2003 Sep-Oct;47(5):777-82.

53. Brauer RJ, Executive Director of the Valley Fever Center for Excellence, VFCE Annual Report 2001-2002.

54. Grant AR, Steinhoff NG, Melick DW. Resectional surgery in pulmonary coccidioidomycosis: a review of 263 cases. In: Ajello L, ed. Coccidioidomycosis: Current clinical and diagnostic status. Miami: Symposia Specialists; 1977: 209-221.

55. Valley Fever Center for Excellence. VFCE Annual Report 2003. Tucson, Arizona: University of Arizona 2003.

56. Valdivia L, Nix D, Wright M, Lindberg E, Fagan T, Lieberman D, Stoffer T, Ampel NM, Galgiani JN. Coccidioidomycosis as a common cause of community-acquired pneumonia. Emerg Infect Dis. 2006 Jun;12(6):958-62.

57. Barnato AE, Sanders GD, Owens DK. Cost-effectiveness of a potential vaccine for Coccidioides immitis. Emerg Infect Dis. 2001 Sep-Oct;7(5):797-806.

58. Chu JH, Feudtner C, Heydon K, Walsh TJ, Zaoutis TE. Hospitalizations for endemic mycoses: a population-based national study. Clin Infect Dis. 2006 Mar 15;42(6):822-5. Epub 2006 Feb 1.

Appendix C: Glossary

This glossary was designed so Valley Fever patients and their families could easily understand the terms they might find in their medical reports. Many definitions include the relevance of the terms to Valley Fever.

Abdominal viscera: Organs in the abdominal cavity, including the stomach, intestines, kidneys, liver and spleen.

Abscess: A localized collection of pus and rotting tissue in bone, organs, or other tissue.

Acute: Having the rapid onset of severe symptoms.

Adenopathy: A disease or enlargement of the glands, particularly the lymph nodes.

Adrenal glands: Two hormone producing glands that are near the top of each kidney.

Alopecia: Loss of scalp or body hair. This can occur with some antifungal treatments.

Alveolus: (pl. Alveoli) Any of the many tiny air sacs within the lungs.

Ambisome: A newer formulation of amphotericin B that tends to have milder side effects.

Amphotericin B: A powerful liquid antifungal drug that has been available since the 1950's. It is famous for its painful side effects and painful delivery through spinal or intravenous injections. In spite of new formulations that may be less toxic, it has been nicknamed "Ampho-Terrible" over the decades and the nickname remains to this day.

Anaphylactic shock: A severe hypersensitivity to a foreign substance (found in drugs or foods, for example) and can lead to potentially deadly loss of blood pressure and breathing problems.

Anaphylaxis: See anaphylactic shock.

Anastomosis: An opening between two spaces or organs that is created by surgery, injury, or disease.

Anemia: Fewer red blood cells circulating in the body than normal, resulting in a decrease of oxygen.

Anergy: The lack of immune system response to a particular substance or infection.

Anicteric: Not jaundiced. See jaundice.

Anorexia: Loss of appetite. When a loss of appetite is caused by a disease or drugs (such as the ones that treat Valley Fever), it should not be confused with anorexia nervosa, a specific psychological disorder.

Anterior: At the front.

Antemortem: Before death.

Antibacterial: Able to kill bacteria or slow their growth. Useful specifically against bacterial infections.

Antibiotic: Literally "anti-life," antibiotics are drugs made to kill microorganisms or act against their growth. When antibiotics are not specified to work against a particular type of organism (fungi, bacteria, viruses, etc.) the term "antibiotic" is usually interpreted to mean "antibacterial antibiotic."

Antibody: A type of protein made by the immune system to attack a specific antigen. Antibodies are not effective at helping patients overcome their coccidioidomycosis, but they can be spotted during laboratory tests and are therefore useful aids for diagnosis.

Antibody-mediated immunity: Immunity based on the production of B cells that produce antibodies. The antibodies that react to *Coccidioides* do not actually protect people, but are very helpful in clinical diagnosis. Contrast this with cell-mediated immunity.

Antifungal: Able to kill fungi or slow their growth. Useful specifically against fungal infections. Only specific antifungal drugs are effective against Valley Fever infections.

Antigen: A foreign substance that can stimulate a specific immune response in the body. Antigens can be toxins or parts of bacteria, cell tissues, or fungi. Antigens can be useful in blood tests, skin tests, or in other testing methods to see if there is an immune response to certain diseases.

Antioxidants: Vitamin A, Vitamin C, lycopene, and a variety of other substances that prevent damage in the body by free radicals.

Arachnoiditis: Inflammation of a part of the membrane around the brain and spinal cord, often caused by surgeries and lumbar puncture (spinal tap) procedures. This can result in extreme and constant pain.

Articular: Joint related.

Arizona flu: A synonym for coccidioidomycosis.

Arthralgia: Joint pain.

Arthritis: Inflammation of joints. This painful ailment can be an unfortunate part of cocci.

Arthroconidium: (pl. arthroconidia) A small reproductive fungal spore. *Coccidioides* arthroconidia are microscopic and easily inhaled. The inhalation of even one arthroconidium is sufficient to cause a Valley Fever infection.

Arthrodesis: See joint fusion.

Arthrospore: See arthroconidium. This term has been entirely replaced with arthroconidium in the recent *Coccidioides* literature.

Asymptomatic: Showing no signs of a disease. Valley Fever was believed to be asymptomatic in 60% of infections, but recent estimates suggest only half of these infections will not have symptoms. The disease is also known to activate years later even in people who did not show symptoms earlier.

Atypical: Not normal.

Auscultate: To listen to the sounds made by internal organs (usually with a stethoscope) to help medical professionals examine a patient.

Autoimmune disease: A process where the body's organs and tissues are considered foreign and attacked by the body's own immune system.

Azole: A type of antifungal drug often given for Valley Fever or other fungal ailments taken orally. Some examples of azole drugs are fluconazole, posaconazole, and itraconazole.

B cell: B lymphocyte:

B lymphocytes: White blood cells that produce antibodies. See antibody-mediated immunity.

Bacterium: (pl. bacteria) Organisms that are single-celled, are prokaryotic (have DNA that is not organized with chromosomes and do not have a nucleus enclosed in a cell membrane) and reproduce by fission. Bacteria can be spherical, rod-shaped, or have various other shapes. They are sometimes considered plants but do not have chlorophyll, the substance that allows some plants to turn sunlight into carbohydrates. Bacteria are responsible for many diseases.

Benign: Not harmful.

Biofilm: A colony of organisms that hold to surfaces (often artificial surfaces, like medical implants) and are resistant to removal by fluid and even some medication.

Biohazard: A microorganism or substance that poses a threat to humans or animals.

Biological agent: A microorganism or toxin that could be used as a biological weapon.

Biological weapon: A microorganism or toxin that is intentionally used to cause harm to humans. *Coccidioides* is regulated as a Select Agent for its potential use by terrorists as a biological weapon.

Biopsy: A sample of tissue from a living body to be examined to assist a diagnosis.

Blastomycosis: A disease caused by an inhaled fungus (*Blastomyces dermatitidis*) that results in a lung infection with possibilities of disseminated illness. Like Valley Fever, it also does not have a vaccine or cure.

Blood-brain barrier: A membrane that surrounds the brain and spinal cord. Drugs to treat meningitis are often chosen based on their ability to penetrate the blood-brain barrier.

Bone scan: An x-ray test using radioactive materials to show areas in the skeleton with issues such as trauma, infections, inflammation, etc.

Bronchi: Plural for bronchus.

Bronchiectasis: A chronic, sometimes permanent expansion of the bronchi due to a lung disease. Consequences of this can be chronic coughing spasms that can produce blood, mucus, and pus. Bronchiectasis can occur due to Valley Fever.

Bronchiole: A subdivision of bronchial passages.

Bronchoalveolar lavage: A treatment to wash the lungs that can aid in diagnosis of diseases, particularly in patients with an immune deficiency.

Bronchoscopy: A medical procedure where a scope is put through the nose or mouth, down the throat, and into the lung to examine the lung and help diagnose various lung diseases. When using a bronchoscopy for Valley Fever testing and diagnosis, a fluid sample may be taken from the lung to be cultured.

Bronchus: (pl bronchi) One of the air passages of the lungs including those coming from the trachea (windpipe).

Calcification: A process where living tissue becomes hardened because it has collected excess calcium.

Carcinoma: A malignant tumor on the epithelium (the surface of skin or organs) that can spread. This is a type of cancer.

Cardiologist: A doctor who specializes in treating the heart.

Catheter: A flexible medical tubing for taking liquid out of an area or putting it in.

Cavity: A space, an area. A cavity could contain organs (like the abdominal cavity) or be a pitted area in an organ due to a lesion.

CD4: Short for "Cluster of Differentiation 4," CD4 is a protein on the surface of certain immune system cells that helps them to function. CD4+ is pronounced as "See Dee Four Positive" and indicates cells that have this protein. CD4+ T lymphocytes help in the fight against Valley Fever.

Cell: The smallest functional structure within an organism.

Cell-mediated immunity: A human ability to fight infections that is independent of antibodies and uses T lymphocytes and phagocytes to fight the infection. Valley Fever is fought by cell-mediated immunity.

Cellular immunity: See cell-mediated immunity.

Central Nervous System (CNS): The spinal cord, spinal nerves, and brain.

Central venous access catheter: A tube that is surgically implanted into a blood vessel to provide intravenous fluid, provide drugs, or take blood samples.

Cerebrospinal Fluid (CSF): The fluid around the brain and spine.

CF: See complement fixation.

Chemotherapy: The use of chemical treatments that are tailored to fight a specific disease in a patient.

Chest cavity: See thoracic cavity.

Chronic: A symptom, disease, or condition that continues or progresses for a long time.

Clearance: The removal of a substance from the body, or the blood or an organ. The proposed "cure" projects for Valley Fever may clear *Coccidioides* from the patients' bodies, which would guarantee the disease could never reactivate. This is also the effect of sterilization.

CM: A common abbreviation in medical journals for coccidioidomycosis. CM can also be used to mean coccidioidal meningitis, and would only refer to that one symptom of Valley Fever in that document. This can make medical literature confusing to readers who only have a partial document (as it might appear on certain web sites that are broken into separate pages), but, the meaning of "CM" in any given document would be explained at the first time it is used.

Cocci: When Valley Fever is a topic of discussion, cocci is short for coccidioidomycosis (the illness) and sometimes used when referring to *Coccidioides* spp. "Cocci" is also used in laboratories to indicate bacteria with a round shape. This can confuse matters for the lay audience seeking Valley Fever information since *Coccidioides* spherules are round fungi, not bacteria.

Coccidia: A protozoan parasite that commonly infects livestock in their intestinal tract, liver, and other organs. Some Internet sites and occasionally even medical documents have mistakenly confused the details of *Coccidia* and *Coccidioides*. In spite of their similar names, they are totally unrelated organisms.

Coccidioidal: Related to *Coccidioides* fungus. As an example, meningitis that is caused by Valley Fever could be called "coccidioidal meningitis."

Coccidioides: The genus of the fungal parasite that causes Valley Fever. When *Coccidioides* is used in a sentence, it can refer to all species from that genus. Example: "*Coccidioides* spores could be inhaled in Arizona, California, and other states in the Southwest."

Coccidioides immitis: Also known as *C. immitis*. This is the soil fungus that can become airborne in the San Joaquin Valley and other endemic regions in California. *C. immitis* and *C. posadasii* are both species from the genus *Coccidioides* and all *Coccidioides* can infect mammals and cause coccidioidomycosis, the infection commonly known as Valley Fever.

Coccidioides posadasii: A species of *Coccidioides* fungus recognized in 2002, previously thought to be a variation of *C. immitis*. It is abbreviated as *C. posadasii* and sometimes called "Non-California *C. immitis*" due to its geographical distribution and its strong similarity to *C. immitis*. It appears in Arizona, Texas, and other places in the United States, as well as in Mexico and Central America and South America.

Coccidioides sp.: This indicates one species from the genus *Coccidioides*, the fungal organism that causes Valley Fever. The "sp." does not specify which species. This term would be used when it is unknown which particular species of *Coccidioides* is the topic of discussion, or when the discussion could refer to either species. Example: "It is dangerous to inhale even one *Coccidioides* sp. spore." Also see the plural *Coccidioides* spp.

Coccidioides spp.: This is a plural term indicating more than one species from the genus *Coccidioides,* a distinction that became necessary when researchers discovered variations in the fungi that cause Valley Fever. Example: "*Coccidioides* spp. cultures should be handled in a lab using Biosafety Level 3 protocols." *Coccidioides* spp. can be abbreviated simply to *Coccidioides* when discussing all species of the same genus. Also see the definitions for *Coccidioides* and *Coccidioides* sp.

Coccidioidin: A solution of *Coccidioides* antigens that does not cause infections but was used as the original Valley Fever skin test.

Coccidioidomycosis: The medical name for the disease commonly called Valley Fever. This is a fungal infection caused by inhaling *C. immitis* or *C. posadasii* spores. It can frequently be characterized by flu-like symptoms, rashes, and joint pains. It can also cause many other destructive, painful, and lethal symptoms, which can make it difficult to diagnose without specific testing. *Coccidioides* can spread from its primary infection in the lungs to affect any part of the body. Coccidioidomycosis is the scientific name for San Joaquin Valley Fever and some of its nicknames are cocci, desert fever, desert rheumatism, Arizona Flu, California's Disease, Posadas' Disease, etc.

Coccidiosis: An infection with the protozoan parasite *Coccidia.* In spite of its similar name, coccidiosis is totally unrelated to coccidioidomycosis.

Community Acquired Pneumonia: Pneumonia that is contracted outside of a hospital.

Complement fixation: A titer test on blood or cerebrospinal fluid to check whether a person has antibodies to *Coccidioides.* Traditional complement fixation titers detect both the earliest (IgM) and later (IgG) antibodies to indicate the body's response to the Valley Fever infection. When used with some newer tests like enzyme immunoassays, the terms "CF titer" or "complement fixing antibodies" often refers only to the IgG antibodies.

Compounding pharmacy: A facility that formulates drugs to a doctor's or pharmacist's specification. This can be different from purchasing pills that have already been manufactured because compounding pharmacies can produce drugs without dyes, change the mix of chemicals, or provide crushed pills in powdered form, for example.

Computed Tomography: A medical procedure that constructs a three-dimensional model from a series of two-dimensional images taken with x-rays at different angles. This is also known as a CT scan and can be used to diagnose a variety of physical conditions.

Concomitant: At the same time. For example, Valley Fever patients with concomitant diabetes often have more severe symptoms.

Congestive heart failure: This is a condition when the heart cannot keep blood circulating sufficiently through the body. This can be life threatening.

Conjunctivitis: Inflammation of the membrane of the eyelids and outer surface of the eye.

Contagious: The ability to spread a disease by direct or indirect contact. Valley Fever is not spread by an infected person's cough but can be spread from direct contact of an open infectious lesion to cuts on another person's skin.

Costochondritis: Inflammation of the cartilage connecting ribs to the sternum, resulting in chest pain. This has been considered similar to pains caused by cocci in medical journals, and patients informed us their costochondritis was diagnosed as a part of their Valley Fever.

Costophrenic: Related to the ribs and diaphragm.

Crackle: Rough sounds that can be heard with a stethoscope. Crackles may indicate pleurisy in the lung.

Cryptococcosis: Infection with *Cryptococcus neoformans*. Cryptococcosis is caused by an inhaled fungus that results in a lung infection with possibilities of disseminated illness. There presently is no vaccine or cure.

CT scan: See computed tomography.

Culture: To grow under laboratory conditions. *Coccidioides* cultures can aid in diagnosis of Valley Fever.

Cure: To a lay audience, a person is cured of a disease when the disease organism is permanently killed and can never return. To a doctor, cure means that an illness' symptoms have completely stopped. The distinction is that the doctors' definition includes diseases that can reactivate like Valley Fever. For example, patients could be declared "cured" of Valley Fever, then relapse years later and die of the disease of which they were supposedly "cured." The lay audience's definition of "cure" actually applies to the definitions for clearance and sterilization.

Cutaneous: Having to do with the skin.

Cyanosis: A bluish tint to the skin and mucous membranes to indicate an inadequate amount of oxygen in the blood.

Cyst: A lesion filled with fluid.

Cytokines: Chemicals released by cells to regulate the immune system.

Cytology: The study of cells.

Cytotoxic: Harmful to living cells.

De novo: From the start, anew.

Debridement: The surgical removal of diseased, dead, foreign, inflamed, or infected tissue from or around a lesion.

Decortication: Removing the outer layer of an organ. Partial decortication of a lung, for example, may be needed if the lung's outer layer became scarred due to a Valley Fever infection and restricts breathing.

Dendritic cell: A special cell that activates T lymphocytes (white blood cells) to fight infections.

Depression: A medical condition where a sense of hopelessness interferes with patients' lives.

Desert fever: A synonym for coccidioidomycosis or Valley Fever.

Desert rheumatism: A synonym for coccidioidomycosis or Valley Fever.

Desiccation: To completely dry up. As one might expect of fungi that live in a desert, *Coccidioides* spp. spores are highly resistant to desiccation.

Diabetes: An illness (often diabetes mellitus) that results in high blood sugar, excess urination, and other problems. Since it is a risk factor for Valley Fever's worst symptoms, patients with diabetes urgently need to know about the dangers of Valley Fever.

Diflucan: Brand name of the antifungal drug fluconazole.

Dimorphic: Having two forms and the ability to change from one to the other. *Coccidioides* spp. is dimorphic because it has a soil form and a parasitic form.

Disarticulation: Separation at the joint. *Coccidioides* arthroconidia become airborne when soil disturbances or wind disarticulate them from the rest of their colony.

Dissemination: The spread of Valley Fever from its site of infection in the lung to other parts of the body through the bloodstream. Valley Fever can disseminate to nearly any organ or body part.

DNA Probe: A diagnostic test that uses genetic material marked with dyes, radioactivity, or enzymes. This material is designed to bond with a specific organism to show whether a person is infected with that organism.

Dysphagia: Difficulty swallowing.

Dysphonia: Difficulty speaking.

Dyspnea: Difficulty breathing.

Ebola: A virus that causes fever, bleeding from every orifice, and shock. It is lethal in up to 90% of patients infected and is so easily transmitted that it is handled in laboratories under Biosafety Level 4 safety protocols (the highest level). To indicate its danger, its safety level is only one step above the Biosafety Level 3 laboratory precautions used when culturing *Coccidioides* spp. or handling objects known or likely to contain *Coccidioides*.

Edema: Tissue swelling from an abnormal increase of fluid in an area.

EIA (Enzyme immunoabsorbent assay or enzyme immunoassay): A type of blood test that measures antibodies.

Electroencephalogram (EEG): A brainwave examination performed with electrodes on the scalp.

Electrocardiogram (EKG or ECG): A test that measures the heart's electrical activity. Also called a cardiograph.

ELISA (Enzyme-linked immunoabsorbent assay): A type of enzyme immunoassay (EIA) blood test. See EIA.

Empirical treatment: Drugs given to a patient based on a doctor's guess about what might help when the cause of the patient's illness has not been proven scientifically.

Empyema: Pus accumulation within a body cavity. When the word "empyema" is used without further description, it refers to pus around the lung in the pleural cavity (thoracic empyema).

Encephalitis: This is the inflammation of the brain itself, as opposed to its lining (the meninges). Encephalitis is sometimes called "Sleeping Sickness" because it creates a sense of apathy and abnormal sleepiness.

Endemic: Related to a specific geographical area, particularly in relation to disease. A disease that is constantly present in a given area is an endemic disease. An endemic area or region is a place where a specific disease causing organism can be found. An endemic area to *Coccidioides* spp. is a place where these fungi grow. See: endemic disease and endemic region.

Endemic disease: A disease that is constantly present in a given area. See our Valley Fever Fundamentals Chapter for the known areas in the United States where the disease Valley Fever is endemic. The areas near the fungal growth are obviously hit the hardest by the disease. Valley Fever is also endemic in parts of Mexico, Central America, and South America.

Endemic region (or endemic area or endemic zone): In relation to Valley Fever, this is a place where *Coccidioides* grows in the soil. The wind can pick up and spread the spores. People and animals can inhale those spores, and the resulting fungal infection is known as Valley Fever. See our Valley Fever Fundamentals Chapter for the areas in the United States where *Coccidioides* grows.

Endobronchial: In the bronchi or bronchial tubes. See bronchus. Endobronchial is synonymous with intrabronchial.

Endocarditis: Inflammation of the inner lining of the heart cavities.

Endocardium: The inner layer of the heart.

Endocrine: See hormone.

Endogenous: From inside. An "endogenous Valley Fever reinfection" would mean the same thing as a "Valley Fever reactivation" because the fungal parasite was already inside the body. Endogenous is the opposite of exogenous.

Endophthalmitis: Inflammation of parts of the inner eye caused by tumors, particles, or fungi.

Endoscope: A thin flexible tube with a camera and a light in it that can be inserted into patient to assist in surgery and diagnosis.

Endospore: A small spore that forms within a parasitic *Coccidioides* spherule. When the parasitic *Coccidioides* spherule reaches maturity, it breaks open to release as many as 1,000 endospores. The presence of endospores in a patient's tissue are considered highly characteristic of Valley Fever so their discovery can lead to a Valley Fever diagnosis if one had not already been made.

Enucleation: Removal, like the surgical removal of a tumor or lesion.

Enzyme: A protein produced by living organisms that assists with chemical reactions in the body.

Enzyme immunoabsorbent assay: See EIA.

Enzyme immunoassay: See EIA.

Eosinophil: A type of white blood cell that responds to malignancies and parasitic infections.

Eosinophilia: An unusually high eosinophil count, which can often be found in people with active Valley Fever or other infections.

Epidemic: A rapidly spreading disease outbreak.

Epidemiologist: A person who studies the causes and control of diseases.

Epidemiology: The medical study of the causes and control of diseases.

Epithelium: The surface layer of skin or an organ.

Equivocal: Unclear or having more than one possible meaning. When used on a laboratory test for Valley Fever, an equivocal result means that the test could not confirm a positive or negative diagnosis.

Erythema: A red rash that is formed as a reaction to some infections, including Valley Fever.

Erythema nodosum: A problem commonly associated with coccidioidomycosis, causing tender red nodules under the skin. It usually occurs on the shins but can appear elsewhere on the body. This inflammatory reaction can occur with arthritic pain and fever at the same time. It occurs more often in women.

Erythema multiforme: A skin condition similar to erythema nodosum but with concentric rings of discoloration around the lesions.

Erythrocyte: A red blood cell.

Erythrocyte Sedimentation Rate (ESR): A test that studies how quickly red blood cells from a patient's blood sample settle at the bottom of a test tube. This can check for inflammation. Also known as a sed rate. A study had shown that 96% of Valley Fever patients with an ESR over 15 mm/hr had disseminated infections. [Source: Crum NF, Wallace MR. Laboratory Values Are Predictive of Disseminated Coccidioidomycosis. Infectious Diseases in Clinical Practice. 13(2):68-72, March 2005.]

Etiology: The cause of an infection or the study of the cause of an infection.

Exogenous: From outside. When people inhale *Coccidioides*, it is an exogenous infection. Exogenous is the opposite of endogenous.

False negative: An incorrect negative test result for a disease when the patient is actually infected with that disease. False negatives are common in Valley Fever patients.

Fibrosis: The buildup of excess fibrous connective material (often scar tissue) in the body.

Filament: A thin thread-like structure of cells. Hyphae from *Coccidioides* spp. are filaments.

Fine Needle Aspiration: The removal of bodily tissue or fluid with a needle for evaluation. Also called a fine needle biopsy. This technique is often less invasive than a surgical biopsy.

Fluconazole: The generic name of the azole drug sold under the brand name Diflucan.

Fomite: Anything that may harbor or transport an infectious organism. *Coccidioides* spores have been transported on cotton, cars, wool, clothing, agricultural produce, and a variety of other materials as fomites to infect patients far outside the endemic areas.

Foot drop: A paralysis or weakness of the toes and ankles that causes the foot or feet to drag when walking.

Free radical: A substance that delivers oxygen to the body in harmful ways, often associated with sickness, stress, immune system problems, and aging.

Fungemia: Fungi circulating in the bloodstream. Also known as fungal sepsis.

Fungicidal: Able to kill fungi.

Fungistatic: Able to slow a fungal infection to the point where it does not worsen. The antifungal drugs used against Valley Fever are said to be fungistatic because it usually appears to be up to the patients' immune systems to determine the outcome of infections. There are also Valley Fever cases where the drugs are not fungistatic because they were unable to prevent the spread and increasing severity of the disease. Some drugs that are said to be fungistatic are also called fungicidal because they can kill fungi under certain conditions, but they may not kill enough fungi to eradicate a specific type of infection completely.

Fungus: (pl. fungi) A simple plant-like organism that has no roots, leaves, stems, or chlorophyll, and reproduces through the use of spores.

Gene: A section of the DNA that indicate how cells should utilize protein.

Gene probe: See DNA probe.

Genetic: Inherited.

Genitourinary tract: The system that includes the sexual organs and the organs (including the kidneys and bladder) that produce, store, and eliminate urine.

Genotype: An organism's genetic structure or the genetic details that allow a particular trait to be expressed.

GP: General practitioner.

General practitioner: A doctor who is not a specialist in any one field but sees patients regularly for a variety of illnesses or medical issues.

Granuloma: An inflammatory lesion that is filled with a variety of cells, some of which are repairing or defending tissue (like immune system cells) and some are destroying tissue. In the medical literature from the 1950's and 1960's, "Coccidioidal granuloma" was a common term for lung lesions caused by Valley Fever.

Granulomatous: Like a granuloma.

Gynecomastia: The abnormal and potentially painful enlargement of male breasts. Sometimes associated with the drug ketoconazole (Nizoral).

Hematology: The study of blood diseases and organs that produce blood.

Hematologist: A doctor specializing in blood diseases and organs that produce blood.

Hematopoietic: Referring to the production of blood or blood cells.

Hemopoiesis: The production of blood or blood cells.

Hemoptysis: Coughing up blood.

Hepatic: Liver related.

Hepatotoxic: Damaging to the liver.

Hepatitis: An inflammation of the liver. While there are some viral diseases that cause liver inflammation (Hepatitis A, B, and C, for example), Valley Fever can also inflame the liver and therefore can be a cause of hepatitis.

Hilar: Related to a hilum.

Hilum: The area that nerves, blood vessels, or bronchi pass through to enter an organ.

Histology: The study of the microscopic detail and function of organs and tissues.

Histopathologist: A physician who studies and diagnoses ailments in tissues, blood, and other bodily fluids. Histopathologists often study suspected tumors.

Histoplasmosis: A disease similar to Valley Fever that is caused by an inhaled fungus (*Histoplasma capsulatum*). It results in a lung infection with possibilities of disseminated illness. Like Valley Fever, it also does not have a vaccine or cure. This fungus is commonly found where bird or bat droppings have accumulated and can be inhaled (including agricultural settings and near building ventilation systems). Histoplasmosis is contracted in many places all over the world. However, it is notably endemic in the soils of the Mississippi and Ohio River valleys, South America, Central America, France, Africa, the Caribbean, and the Far East. [Source: MDAinternet.com] Histoplasmosis, blastomycosis, and other fungal ailments often produce similar symptoms to Valley Fever.

HIV (human immunodeficiency virus): The virus that causes Acquired Immune Deficiency Syndrome (AIDS). This virus harms the immune system, allowing the syndrome to occur.

Hormone: A secretion from an organ or bodily tissue that is designed to have an effect on another organ or organs.

Host: The organism that a parasite takes its nutrition from. When people have Valley Fever, they are hosts to *Coccidioides*.

Human genome: All the DNA found in humans.

Humoral: In Valley Fever, this usually relates to the production of antibodies. See: Antibody-mediated immunity. Humoral can also mean "related to hormones and bodily fluid."

Humoral immunity: See antibody-mediated immunity.

Hydrocephalus: Excess pressure from spinal fluid on the brain.

Hypercalcemia: An abnormally high amount of calcium in the blood. It is often associated with cancer but also can be associated with Valley Fever. Hypercalcemia can lead to a variety of problems including heart arrhythmia (abnormal rhythm), osteoporosis (loss of bone mass), and kidney stones. If the calcium level remains abnormally high in the blood it could lead to death.

Hyperesthesia: An abnormal and possibly painful increase in sensitivity to touch, sound, taste, etc.

Hyperglycemia: A state of abnormally high blood sugar, often due to diabetes. Diabetes presents enhanced risks for Valley Fever's most severe symptoms.

Hyperplastic: An abnormal increase in the number of cells in an organ or tissue. This can cause an abnormal size increase for the organ.

Hypha: (pl. hyphae) A fibrous tube-like thread produced by a fungus. *Coccidioides* produces hyphae to grow in the soil and occasionally (but not normally) in human hosts.

Hypokalemia: Abnormally low blood potassium, which can be lethal in severe cases.

Icteric: See jaundice.

ID doctor: See infectious disease doctor.

Idiopathic: From an unknown cause. Valley Fever symptoms are often considered idiopathic until the correct diagnosis is made.

IgG (Immunoglobulin G antibodies): These are the antibodies that appear several weeks and months into Valley Fever cases to indicate an ongoing or previous infection.

IgM (Immunoglobulin M antibodies): These are the antibodies that appear soonest in a Valley Fever infection, often after the first few weeks. Their presence tends to indicate a new or ongoing infection.

Immune: Protected from a disease. While a lay audience would interpret this to mean total protection with no possibility of future problems from the disease, this is not always the case. People who have been proven to have an immune resistance to Valley Fever have still experienced relapses, infections from additional spores, and even chronic, debilitating, and fatal cases.

Immune System: The cells and organs that fight against diseases and infections within the body.

Immunize: To make immune.

Immunoassay: A laboratory testing method that checks to see if antibodies react with an antigen.

Immunocompetent: Having a normal, healthy immune system. Most people who contract Valley Fever are immunocompetent.

Immunocompromised: Having a weakened immune system, possibly due to specific medical conditions or as a result of medical treatments.

Immunodeficiency: Same as immunocompromised. See immunocompromised.

Immunodiffusion: A blood test to find antibodies to a specific antigen by placing them together and seeing whether they react chemically.

Immunomodulation: Intentional changes to the immune system's normal abilities. These may ultimately be able to help Valley Fever patients who suffer with anergy.

Immunosuppression: A reduction of the immune system's abilities. Often this occurs due to medical treatments with drugs like corticosteroids or those used during organ transplantation.

In vitro: In laboratory conditions, not within a body.

In vivo: Within the body. In vivo testing occurs in laboratory animals or in human volunteers, and is considered more valuable than in vitro testing.

Inconclusive: Uncertain. An inconclusive test does not have any results that can confirm a positive or negative diagnosis.

Incurable: Not able to be completely healed by current medicine. Since treatment does not eliminate all *Coccidioides* spores in the body and they can reactivate after becoming dormant, Valley Fever is presently an incurable disease.

Indeterminate: Unclear or having more than one possible meaning. When used on a laboratory test for Valley Fever, an indeterminate result means that the test could not confirm a positive or negative diagnosis.

Infection: A medical condition caused by an invasive disease organism within the body.

Infectious disease doctor: A medical specialist in diseases caused by microscopic organisms.

Infiltrate: An infection that penetrates the healthy tissue around it. Valley Fever infiltrates in the lung can produce a "road map" like appearance of scarring on x-rays.

Inflammation: The presence of abnormal redness, swelling, pain, decreased blood flow, loss of function, and warmth at a specific part or parts of the body. This is a general symptom that could be produced by many different causes.

Inflammatory: Causing inflammation.

Inoculum: The organism or tissues that start disease processes or the material that can be used as a vaccine to provide a specific type of immunity.

Internist: A doctor who is not a surgeon but specializes in the treatment of diseases that affect internal organs.

Intrabronchial: In the bronchi or bronchial tubes. See bronchus. Intrabronchial is synonymous with endobronchial.

Intrathecal: Between the brain and the spinal cord's lining. This is often where amphotericin B treatments may need to be delivered so they may penetrate the blood-brain barrier more completely and quickly.

Intravenous (IV): Into a vein. Sometimes antifungal treatments are provided intravenously.

Intraocular: In the eye.

Invasive: The description of a disease organism that spreads to healthy tissue. Also used to describe a medical procedure (such as surgery or testing) that requires something to enter a part of the body by puncture or incision.

Iridocyclitis: Inflammation of the iris and its controlling muscles.

Itraconazole: The generic name of an azole drug sold under the brand name Sporanox.

Jaundice: Having yellowed skin and eyes because of excess biliruben (a pigment in bile) in the blood. Jaundice often indicates a disease process.

Joint fusion: Permanent surgical prevention of a joint's mobility so the bones will grow together into one mass. This is usually done to prevent joint pain or the progress of a disease. Also known as arthrodesis.

Keratotic ulcers: Lesions with a wartlike surface.

Ketoconazole: The generic name of an azole drug sold under the brand name Nizoral.

Laproscope: A thin fiber optic tube with a camera (a type of endoscope) that can be inserted into patients to allow doctors to perform surgery or diagnose illness in the patient.

Larynx: Voice box.

Latex agglutination: In Valley Fever, it is a test that finds IgM antibodies.

Legionella: A bacterium that can cause Legionnaires' Disease, an illness that has many symptoms in common with Valley Fever. Some patients with Valley Fever have been misdiagnosed with this bacterial infection.

Lesion: A localized area of diseased or abnormally changed tissue. Blisters, cysts, nodules, and ulcers are examples of lesions.

Leucocytes: A general term for the parts of the blood that defend the body against infections. Also known as white blood cells.

Leucocytosis: An abnormal elevation of the white blood cell count in blood. This may indicate an infection.

Leucopenia: An abnormal decreased presence of white blood cells.

Lipids: Organic compounds including fat, wax, and oil that do not dissolve in water. New formulations of amphotericin B that use lipids tend to have milder side effects.

Lobe: A natural division of part of an organ, such as the liver, brain, or lung.

Lobectomy: Surgery to remove a lobe of an organ, commonly the lung in Valley Fever patients.

Local anesthesia: Medication to temporarily numb sensation in a localized part of the body to protect patients from the pain of surgery at that spot.

Lumbar puncture: Placement of a needle into the cerebrospinal fluid (CSF) to collect some of the fluid for testing or to insert medication. Also known as a spinal tap.

Lymph: The clear fluid in bodily tissues that contains white blood cells.

Lymphadenopathy: Abnormal and chronic swelling of the lymph nodes.

Lymphatic system: Lymph nodes, bone marrow, and the organs and vessels that carry lymph.

Lymphedema: Swelling in a limb due to accumulation of excess fluid, often due to radiation treatments near a lymph node, tumors near a lymph node, or because a lymph node was surgically removed.

Lymphocyte: A type of white blood cell that is either a B Cell or T Cell.

Lymph nodes: Small bean-shaped glands that filter infectious microorganisms and cancer cells in the lymph.

Lysin: An antibody or other substance that can produce lysis.

Lysis: Destruction or decomposition of cells due to the rupture of the cell membranes or wall.

Lytic: Causing lysis. Often this refers to lytic lesions, where healthy cells are being destroyed within the lesion.

Macrophage: A large white blood cell that is a phagocyte (it defends the body by surrounding, destroying, and removing foreign substances).

Malignant: Life threatening. Also applied to cancerous tumors that destroy the tissue they are in and may spread to new tissue through the blood.

Malignancy: A cancerous growth. Lesions caused by Valley Fever have frequently been misdiagnosed as malignancies.

Mediastinal: Related to the mediastinum.

Mediastinal lymphadenopathy: Inflammation or disease of the mediastinal lymph nodes.

Mediastinoscope: An optical scope placed through a surgical incision above the patient's sternum, useful for obtaining biopsies.

Mediastinum: The space in the middle of the chest between both pleural sacs (containing the lungs).

Membrane: A protective layer of tissue around some organs, surfaces, and cells.

Meninges: The three membranes that form a protective outer layer around the brain and spinal cord.

Meningioma: A tumor of the meninges that can cause headaches and other problems due to pressure on the brain.

Meningitis: Inflammation of the lining of the brain and spinal cord, the meninges. Although some forms of meningitis are contagious, meningitis from coccidioidomycosis is not. It is, however, considered the worst and most lethal form of *Coccidioides* infection.

Metastasis: To spread by blood, lymph, or organ surfaces to another part of the body. While cancer is known to metastasize, *Coccidioides* is said to disseminate. See dissemination.

Micrometer: One millionth of a meter.

Micron: An old term for micrometer.

Miliary: Having the appearance of small, close lesions that often resemble millet seeds.

Mold: Fungal growth on decaying organic matter.

Morbidity: Illness.

Morphology: The biological study of an organism's structure.

Mortality: Death.

MRI (Magnetic Resonance Imaging): An electromagnetic scan that can create clear images of internal bodily structures to assist a diagnosis. See tomography.

Mucopurulent: Containing mucus and pus.

Mucosa: A mucous membrane.

Mucosal: Relating to a mucous membrane.

Mucous: Covered with, making, or resembling mucus.

Mucous membrane: The lining of an internal surface of a cavity that leads outside the body and has glands to produce mucus.

Mucus: A slimy liquid that protects and lubricates bodily surfaces.

Myalgia: Muscle pain.

Mycelium: (pl. mycelia) A mass of hyphae (fibrous tube-like fungal structures). *Coccidioides* colonies are known to form mycelia in the soil.

Mycology: The study of fungi.

Mycosis: (pl. mycoses) Disease caused by a fungus.

Mycotic: Relating to a mycosis.

Myocarditis: Inflammation of the heart's muscular wall.

Necrosis: The process of cellular breakdown in dying bodily tissue.

Necrotic: Dying, as applied to tissue. Bodily tissue that is rotting could be called necrotic.

Negative: A test result that says a test could not find the infection it was looking for, and indicates that the patient does not have the infection. Also see false negative.

Neoplasm: Abnormal tissue growth that may either be benign (neither spreading nor dangerous) or malignant (both spreading and dangerous) and does not perform a bodily function. Synonymous with tumor.

Nephric: Kidney related.

Nephrogenic systemic fibrosis (NSF): An excessive buildup of fibrous tissue throughout the body that can lead to limitation of movement, paralysis, and death.

Nephrotoxic: Damaging to the kidneys.

Nervous system: The spinal cord, brain, and nerves.

Neurologist: A medical doctor specializing in brain and nervous system diseases.

Neurology: Study of the nervous system.

Neuropathy: A general term about changes and problems in the peripheral nervous system (the nerves that connect to the Central Nervous System).

Neutropenia: A reduction of neutrophils in the blood, leading to an immunocompromised state.

Neutrophil: A type of white blood cell.

Nizoral: Name brand of the antifungal drug Ketoconazole.

Nodule: A lump or collection of cells and tissue.

Non-endemic: Areas that do not have a high prevalence of a particular disease or the disease causing organism.

Ommaya reservoir: A surgically implanted dome-shaped device with a catheter. It is placed near the brain to allow repeated medical access to cerebrospinal fluid (CSF), either to drain CSF, test CSF, or to put medication into the CSF.

Oncology: The study of cancer. Cancer misdiagnoses are common with Valley Fever.

Oropharynx: The cavity formed at the back of the mouth by the pharynx.

Orphan disease: A disease that does not have a cure, is not adequately treatable, and qualifies for orphan drug status. See orphan drug.

Orphan drug: A term used by the FDA to describe drugs that are used to treat diseases that affect less than 200,000 people. This term is used for grant appeals for medical research projects.

Orthostatic: Relating to proper upright posture.

Osteomyelitis: An inflammation of the bone by organisms causing a buildup of pus. It can spread from one bone to another or remain localized and may ultimately require limbs to be amputated due to the damage. Osteomyelitis is one of the most devastating conditions that can be caused by coccidioidomycosis.

Otolaryngology: The study of the ear, nose, and throat.

Otomycosis: A fungal infection of the outer ear canal.

Palsy: Muscle paralysis, often associated with tremors.

Paracentesis: Fluid removal from the abdomen with a needle or tube.

Paraparesis: Weakness or partial paralysis affecting the legs.

Parasite: An animal, plant, or microorganism that takes nutrients from another species (the host).

Paravertebral: Around the backbone/vertebral column.

Paresthesia: An abnormal sensation like numbness, burning, tingling, or increased sensitivity, but without an apparent cause.

Pathogen: A microorganism that can cause a disease.

Pathology: The study of disease.

Pathophysiology: The study of the effects of injury or disease on the body.

PCP: A common abbreviation for "primary care physician."

Percutaneous: Through the skin, as in a percutaneous injection.

Pericardiocentesis: Removal of fluid around the heart.

Pericardium: The sack around the heart.

Peritoneum: The membrane that lines the abdominal cavity and covers the abdominal viscera.

Peritonitis: Inflammation of the peritoneum. This often causes pain, vomiting, and constipation.

PET scan (Positron Emission Tomography scan): A specialized imaging test that studies tissues and organs using radioactive materials that are injected into the patient.

Phagocyte: A cell that can surround and digest microorganisms, cell debris, and other particles in the body. These are a part of the cell-mediated immune response and include macrophages and some lymphocytes.

Pharynx: The passage that includes the nasal cavity and the back of the mouth to the esophagus.

Phenotype: How an organism looks and functions as a result of its environment and its genetics (genotype).

Phlegmon: Inflammation and pus in connective tissue.

Pituitary gland: A gland that regulates hormones and controls other glands that produce hormones.

Plasma: The liquid part of the blood that contains antibodies and other materials. Antibodies found in the plasma can indicate infections.

Platelet: A blood cell that enables clotting.

Pleura: Membranes around the lungs.

Pleural cavity: The lungs' area within the chest.

Pleural sac: The cavity or pouch containing the lung.

Pleural effusion: A condition of excess fluid in the pleural cavity.

Pleurisy: See pleuritis.

Pleuritis: Inflammation of the membranes around the lung and the lung cavity.

Pneumonia: Inflammation of the lungs.

Pneumothorax: An abnormal presence of air in the pleural cavity (around the lungs) that can collapse the lung.

Posaconazole: A new and powerful azole drug sold under the brand name Noxafil.

Positive: A disease test that says the patient is infected with that disease.

Posterior: At the back.

Postmortem: After death.

Prognosis: A predictive statement about the possible consequences of a medical condition.

Prognostic: Useful to predict the outcome of a disease.

Protozoa: Single-celled organisms that are among the simplest to be found in the animal kingdom. Some feed on bacteria and others may act as parasites.

Pruritis: A strong itching sensation.

Pulmonary: Relating to the lungs.

Pulmonary fibrosis: Lung scarring.

Pulmonologist: A doctor who specializes in lung care.

Purulent: Causing the production of pus or containing pus.

Pustule: A blister (bubble of tissue) on the skin with pus inside.

Pyogenic: Producing pus.

Quantitative: Indicating the measurable amount of something. Complement fixation titers are quantitative because they can indicate the amount of antibodies to *Coccidioides* found in a sample. Sometimes this quantitative information can be used to judge the severity of an illness.

Qualitative: Descriptive. Indicating a distinguishing feature. Qualitative tests are used on patients so doctors can answer the question "what is this organism?" when they test to see if a person has an infection. Skin tests for Valley Fever are qualitative because they can show that a person has been previously infected (people who test positive have a reaction to the *Coccidioides* antigen), but these tests do not show how severe the infection was before or how severe the infection is now.

Quiescent: Not active.

Radiculopathy: Disease at the roots of spinal nerves.

Radiologist: A doctor specializing in the imaging studies such as MRIs, x-rays, etc.

Radiology: The use of medical imaging techniques (x-rays, MRIs, CT scans, etc.) to evaluate medical conditions.

Reagent: A substance that causes a chemical reaction. The Valley Fever skin test reagents were named coccidioidin and spherulin.

Recombinant DNA: The creation of specific DNA arrangements, often to create new medicines or tests.

Reference interval: A type of response to a test that occurred in a specifically controlled group. When testing for *Coccidioides*, this usually refers to the type of response a lab is likely to see when a test has a negative result.

Renal: Kidney related.

Resection: Complete or partial surgical removal of an organ or tissue.

Rheumatism: A painful inflammation that commonly affects muscles and joints but can go into organs such as the heart. Cocci has been known to cause rheumatism.

Rift Valley Fever: A mosquito-borne virus that is native to the Middle East. Despite having "Valley Fever" in its name, it is not related to coccidioidomycosis (aka "San Joaquin Valley Fever").

Roentgenogram: A picture made as the result of an x-ray test.

Roentgenograph: An outdated but occasionally used term for a roentgenogram.

San Joaquin Valley Fever: See coccidioidomycosis.

Saprobe: An organism that consumes decaying animal or plant matter. When a *Coccidioides* colony lives in the soil, it can be called saprobic. Some saprobes feed on material in stagnant water, but this does not apply to *Coccidioides*.

Saprophyte: See saprobe.

Sarcoidosis: A disease of unknown cause that creates lesions that are similar to Valley Fever. Steroid treatments appear to be safer for patients with this disease than for those with Valley Fever.

Scans: Images of internal bodily structures to aid in the diagnosis of medical conditions.

Sclera: The white of the eye.

Sed Rate: See erythrocyte sedimentation rate.

Select Agent: A general term from the CDC's "Select Agent List" to describe toxins or organisms that can be considered an incredible threat to public health. Select Agents are federally regulated in the Antiterrorism and Effective Death Penalty Act of 1996 and the Public Health Security and Bioterrorism Preparedness and Response Act of 2002.

Sepsis: An infection and destruction of body tissue by disease-causing organisms (like bacteria or fungi).

Septic: Related to sepsis, a decomposition of cells due to microorganisms.

Septic shock: A widespread septic infection in the bloodstream accompanied with circulation failures, leading to decreased blood flow, organ failure, and potentially death. This is an infrequently recognized but serious complication of Valley Fever.

Sequela: (pl. sequelae) Any disorder that is a consequence of a previous disease or injury. Scarring from Valley Fever lesions with a permanent decrease in lung capacity can be called coccidioidal sequelae.

Serology: Blood testing for antigens or antibodies.

Serologic: Related to serology.

Serum: (pl. sera) The clear portion of a liquid. Blood serum is plasma without clotting elements and can be useful for antibody testing.

Shock: A circulatory system failure resulting in decreased blood flow, often caused by illness or an injury.

Shunt: A catheter designed to link two parts of the body.

Side effects: Medical complications caused by a medical treatment.

Sinus: A depression on an organ's surface, as Valley Fever's pus-filled lesions can leave after they drain. The term sinus also refers to natural spaces within organs and bones, such as the nasal sinuses.

SOB: An abbreviation for "shortness of breath," a common Valley Fever symptom.

Soft tissue: Material in the body such as nerves, fat, muscle, tendons and other tissues that support and connect bones and other organs within the body.

Somnolent: Sleepy.

Spherule: A round-shaped form of *Coccidioides* that arthroconidia can become when within an animal or human body. Spherules are parasites and can produce a multitude of endospores.

Spherulin: A Valley Fever skin test that uses *Coccidioides* antigens from the spherule form of the fungus.

Spinal cord: A portion of the central nervous system directly below the brain and through the spinal column that sends and receives nerve signals to and from the brain.

Spinal tap: The common term for a lumbar puncture procedure. See lumbar puncture.

Spirometry: Testing to measure the volume of air the lung can inhale and exhale.

Spleen: An internal organ near the stomach that produces immune system cells.

Sporanox: Name brand of the antifungal drug itraconazole.

Spore: A small reproductive body (often from bacteria or fungi) that is capable of resisting great heat and dehydration and can grow into a new organism.

Sporangia: Structures of lower fungi (Zygomycetes) unrelated to *Coccidioides* that produce new spores.

Sputum: Material that is spit from a patient. It can contain saliva and other material from the mouth, throat and lungs.

Sternum: The flat bone between the ribs and directly above the solar plexus. Also called the breastbone.

Sterilize: To completely remove microorganisms. A cure that would prevent reactivation of Valley Fever would sterilize *Coccidioides* from the body.

Sterilization: See sterilize.

Subpleural: Below the membrane that lines the pleural cavity, the space within the chest that holds the lungs.

Susceptible: Able to be infected. When epidemiologists talk about people who are "susceptible" to Valley Fever, they refer to people who have not contracted Valley Fever yet.

Symptoms: Signs of an illness.

Systemic: Affecting the entire body.

T cell: T lymphocyte.

T lymphocytes: Types of white blood cells that can control the body's ability to recognize and attack Valley Fever and many other infections as a part of cell-mediated immunity.

Tenosynovitis: Inflammation of the tendon sheaths, causing joint pain.

Thoracentesis: Removal of fluid from the chest cavity with a needle. This procedure can be done for testing or treatment for a patient.

Thoracic cavity: The area within the rib cage between the diaphragm and the neck. It includes the heart and lungs. Also known as the chest cavity.

Thoracic viscera: Organs in the upper body (thoracic cavity) and including the lungs and heart.

Thoracoscope: A medical fiber optic tube (endoscope) with lighting and camera technology designed to be surgically inserted into the chest cavity. It aids in diagnostic and surgical procedures, such as biopsies and video-assisted thoracic surgery.

Thoracoscopic surgery: Surgery using a thoracoscope.

Thoracotomy: The surgical opening of the chest cavity. Video-assisted thoracic surgery can sometimes be a less invasive option. A thoracotomy typically is performed for Valley Fever patients before a lobectomy or resection of one or both lungs.

Thorax: The part of the torso between the neck and the abdomen.

Thrombocytosis: The presence of excess platelets in the blood.

Thyroid gland: A gland that regulates metabolism, hormones, and the immune system.

Tinnitus: Buzzing or ringing in the ears.

Tissue: A collection of similar bodily cells and materials that are connected as a part of the structure of an organism and work together to perform a specific function.

Titer: A titer is a test to find how much dilution is required for a patient's blood serum not to show any Valley Fever antibodies. When a blood sample is taken, the serum (the clear part of the blood with white and red blood cells taken out) is mixed with a saline solution and then tested. If the VF test is positive (shows that cocci antibodies are still there) it is diluted by half again.

This happens again and again until the cocci test is negative, meaning the serum is so diluted that no antibodies can be found. A titer that is written as "1:8" is read as "one to eight." To say someone has a titer of 1:8 means the mixture could be considered to be one part serum and eight parts solution before the test could become negative. A titer is considered lower when it is less diluted (1:4 is lower than 1:8) and higher when it uses more solution (1:128 is higher than 1:32). Medical sources routinely consider titers of 1:8 and above to be serious. Dissemination is especially common above 1:16. Patients with high titers and dissemination are usually treated with antifungal medication. A low titer can mean the immune system isn't reacting strongly (either due to immune problems or the VF attack wasn't as severe as it could have been) and a high titer can mean the immune system was reacting very strongly (indicating that the VF infection was severe or the immune system just produced many *Coccidioides* antibodies). Regardless of one's immune health, these antibodies are actually useless to help the body fight the disease. They are helpful in diagnosis because the antibodies are easier to spot in the blood than the fungus itself. Some people have no titers detectable even while the disease is at its worst (and even when they do not have a compromised immune system) and others may show high titers while they outwardly appear to be healthy. Even with that consideration, the correlation of a high titer with severe Valley Fever in humans is common and backed up by decades of medical research. The correlation is not very strong in dogs' titer tests.

Tomography: A testing science that constructs detailed images of internal body structures by taking multiple cross sectional images of the internal body structures. Examples of tests that use tomography include PET scans, CT scans, MRI scans, ultrasounds, and other tests.

Trachea: The windpipe.

Trauma: An injury or wound.

Tube precipitin: A test that can find IgM antibodies for coccidioidomycosis.

Tumor: See neoplasm.

Ulcer: A lesion on the surface of the skin or organ that features pus, inflammation, and necrosis (death) of tissue.

Ultrasound: A test that uses high frequency waves to produce images of structures within the body.

Unilateral: On one side, often in reference to pairs of organs. For example, only one lung would be inflamed in a patient with unilateral pneumonia.

Urinalysis: Laboratory testing of urine.

Urinary tract: The entire passage, from the kidney to the external opening of the urethra, from which urine is produced and eliminated.

Urologist: A doctor specializing in medical conditions of the genitourinary tract.

Vaccine: A substance that stimulates the body's immune response to prevent or reduce the severity of a specific type of infection.

Valley Fever: The more common term for "San Joaquin Valley Fever" and coccidioidomycosis. See coccidioidomycosis.

Vasculitis: Inflammation of blood or lymph vessels.

Ventricle: A chamber within the body or an organ, such as the brain's four ventricles that are filled with cerebrospinal fluid or the heart's two ventricles that pump blood.

Ventriculoperitoneal shunt: A specific type of catheter placement that is often used when a patient is being treated for meningitis. The purpose is to use a shunt inserted in the skull to send excess fluid from a ventricle of the brain to the peritoneum (within the abdomen) to reduce the potential for excess pressure on the brain.

Verrucose ulcers: Wartlike outgrowths on the surface of organs and skin.

VF: Shorthand for Valley Fever that is very common on the Internet.

Vfend: Name brand of the antifungal drug voriconazole.

Video-assisted thoracic surgery (also known as video assisted thoracotomy or VAT): Use of a thoracoscope and tube-inserted surgical devices to remove lesions or perform surgeries that otherwise might require the opening of the chest cavity.

Virulence: The degree of capability of a microorganism to cause illness. *Coccidioides* is the most virulent fungus known to man and is regulated by antiterrorism laws.

Virus: Genetic material with a protein coat that can cause infections.

Viscera: Organs in cavities of the body. See thoracic viscera and abdominal viscera.

Vitrectomy: Removal of all or part of the gel-filled body of the eye and its replacement with a saline solution, as may be necessary in some Valley Fever eye infections.

Voriconazole: The generic name of an azole drug sold under the brand name Vfend.

White blood cells: Parts of the blood that defend the body against infections. Also known as leucocytes.

X-ray: A type of electromagnetic radiation that doctors use to create images of internal bodily structures.

Bibliography

1.   Ader R. Conditioned immunomodulation: Research needs and directions. Brain Behav Immun 2003 Feb;17(1 Suppl):51-7.

2.   Adler-Moore J, Proffitt RT. AmBisome: liposomal formulation, structure, mechanism of action and pre-clinical experience. J Antimicrob Chemother. 2002 Feb;49 Suppl 1:21-30.

3.   Alberda C, Gramlich L, Meddings J, Field C, McCargar L, Kutsogiannis D, Fedorak R, Madsen K. Effects of probiotic therapy in critically ill patients: a randomized, double-blind, placebo-controlled trial. Am J Clin Nutr. 2007 Mar;85(3):816-23.

4.   American College of Radiology. One Size Does Not Fit All: Reducing Risks from Pediatric CT. ACR Bulletin. 2001 Feb;57(2):20-23.

5.   Ampel NM. Coccidioidomycosis in persons infected with HIV-1. Ann N Y Acad Sci. 2007 Sep;1111:336-42. Epub 2007 Mar 15.

6.   Ampel NM. The complex immunology of human coccidioidomycosis. Ann N Y Acad Sci. 2007 Sep;1111:245-58. Epub 2007 Mar 15.

7.   Ampel NM, Dols CL, Galgiani JN. Coccidioidomycosis during human immunodeficiency virus infection: results of a prospective study in a coccidioidal endemic area. Am J Med. 1993 Mar;94(3):235-40.

8.   Answers.com. Free Radical. www.answers.com/topic/free-radical Accessed 2007 April 4.

9.   Antony SJ, Jurczyk P, Brumble L. Successful use of combination antifungal therapy in the treatment of coccidioides meningitis. J Natl Med Assoc. 2006 Jun;98(6):940-2.

10.   Arsura EL. The association of age and mortality in coccidioidomycosis [letter]. J Am Geriatr Soc 1997;45:532-3.

11.   Arsura EL, Caldwell J, Johnson R, Einstein H, Welch G, Talbot R, Affentranger H. Coccidioidomycosis epidemic of 1991: Epidemiologic features.   In: Einstein HE, CatanzaroA, eds.   Coccidioidomycosis. Proceedings of the 5th International Conference on Coccidioidomycosis. Stanford University, 24-27 August, 1994. Washington DC: National Foundation for Infectious Diseases, 1996: 98-107.

12.   Arup Labs. Coccidioides Antibody. ARUP's Guide to Clinical Laboratory Testing.   http://www.aruplab.com/guides/clt/tests/clt_a180.jsp#1059843 Accessed 2006 June 22.

13.   Arup Labs. User's Guides. http://www.aruplab.com/guides/ug/tests/ugc.jsp Accessed 2006 July 13.

14.   Arup Labs. User's Guides. Coccidioides Antibodies Panel, Serum by CF, ID, ELISA. http://www.aruplab.com/guides/ug/tests/0050588.jsp   Accessed 2006 July 16.

15.   Arup Labs. User's Guides. Coccidioides immitis Identification by DNA Probe.   http://www.aruplab.com/guides/ug/tests/0062225.jsp   Accessed 2006 July 13.

16.   Arup Labs. User's Guides. Coccidioides immitis Identification by ID. http://www.aruplab.com/guides/ug/tests/0050183.jsp   Accessed 2006 July 16.

17.   Asgari M, Owrang A.   Results of skin test surveys for systemic mycoses in Iran. Mycopathol Mycol Appl 1970;41(1):91-106.

18.   Assi MA, Binnicker MJ, Wengenack NL, Deziel PJ, Badley AD. Disseminated coccidioidomycosis in a liver transplant recipient with negative serology: use of polymerase chain reaction. Liver Transpl. 2006 Aug;12(8):1290-2.

19.   Barnato AE, Sanders GD, Owens DK.   Cost-effectiveness of a potential vaccine for Coccidioides immitis. Emerg Infect Dis. 2001 Sep-Oct;7(5):797-806.

20.   Bellin HJ, Bhagavan BS. Coccidioidomycosis of the prostate gland. Report of a case and review of the literature. Arch Pathol. 1973 Aug;96(2):114-7.

21.   Blair JE. Coccidioidomycosis in patients who have undergone transplantation. Ann N Y Acad Sci. 2007 Sep;1111:365-76. Epub 2007 Mar 15

22.   Blair JE, Balan V, Douglas DD, Hentz JG.   Incidence and prevalence of coccidioidomycosis in patients with end-stage liver disease. Liver Transpl. 2003 Aug;9(8):843-50.

23.   Blitzer A, Lawson W.   Fungal infections of the nose and paranasal sinuses. Part I. Otolaryngol Clin North Am 1993 Dec;26(6):1007-35.

24.   Bouza E, Dreyer JS, Hewitt WL, Meyer RD. Coccidioidal meningitis. An analysis of thirty-one cases and review of the literature. Medicine (Baltimore) 1981 May;60(3):139-72 citing Hart PD, Russell E, Remington JS: The compromised host and infection. II. Deep fungal infection. J Infect Dis., 120: 169, 1969.

25.   Brajtburg J, Bolard J. Carrier effects on biological activity of amphotericin B. Clin Microbiol Rev. 1996 Oct;9(4):512-31.

26.   Brauer RJ, Executive Director of Valley Fever Center for Excellence (VFCE). VFCE Annual Report 2001-2002. Tucson, Arizona: University of Arizona 2002.

27.   Brauer RJ, personal communication.

28.   Bulmer GS. Medical mycology. Chicago: Year Book Medical Publishers, Inc., 1979: Introduction.

29.   Busowski JD, Safdar A. Treatment for coccidioidomycosis in pregnancy? Postgrad Med. 2001 Mar;109(3):76-7.

30.   Caldwell JW, Johnson RH. The economic impact of coccidioidomycosis in Kern County, California, 1991-1993. In: Einstein HE, Catanzaro A, eds. Coccidioidomycosis. Proceedings of the 5th International Conference on Coccidioidomycosis. Stanford University, 24-27 August, 1994. Washington, DC. National Foundation for Infectious Diseases; 1996: 88-97.

31.   Caraway NP, Fanning CV, Stewart JM, Tarrand JJ, Weber KL. Coccidioidomycosis osteomyelitis masquerading as a bone tumor. A report of 2 cases. Acta Cytol. 2003 Sep-Oct;47(5):777-82.

32.   Cardone JS, Vinson R, Anderson LL. Coccidioidomycosis: the other great imitator. Cutis 1995 Jul;56(1):33-6.

33.   Carrada-Bravo T. Coccidioidomycosis in children. Bol Med Hosp Infant Mex 1989 Jul;46(7):507-14. Abstract translated at Pubmed.

34.   Castanon-Olivares LR, Guerena-Elizalde D, Gonzalez-Martinez MR, Licea-Navarro AF, Gonzalez-Gonzalez GM, Aroch-Calderon. Molecular identification of coccidioides isolates from mexican patients. Ann N Y Acad Sci. 2007 Oct;1111:326-35. Epub 2007 Mar 7.

35.   Catanzaro A. Pulmonary mycosis in pregnant women. Chest. 1984 Sep;86(3 Suppl):14S-18S.

36.   Catanzaro A, Cloud GA, Stevens DA, Levine BE, Williams PL, Johnson RH, Rendon A, Mirels LF, Lutz JE, Holloway M, Galgiani JN. Safety, tolerance, and efficacy of posaconazole therapy in patients with nonmeningeal disseminated or chronic pulmonary coccidioidomycosis. Clin Infect Dis. 2007 Sep 1;45(5):562-8. Epub 2007 Jul 23.

37.   Catanzaro A, Einstein H, Levine B, Ross JB, Schillaci R, Fierer J, Friedman PJ. Ketoconazole for treatment of disseminated coccidioidomycosis. Ann Intern Med 1982 Apr;96(4):436-40.

38.   CDC. Coccidioidomycosis--Arizona, 1990-1995. MMWR Morb Mortal Wkly Rep. 1996 Dec 13;45(49):1069-73.

39.   CDC. Notification of Exclusion. Select Agent Program. Centers for Disease Control and Prevention. http://www.cdc.gov/od/sap/sap/exclusion.htm Accessed 2007 Dec 06.

40.   CDC. Press Release: Hand Hygiene in Healthcare Settings. Accessible online at http://www.cdc.gov/handhygiene/pressrelease.htm 2002 Oct 25.

41.   CDC. Provisional cases of selected notifiable diseases, United States, weeks ending December 29, 2007, and December 30, 2006 (52nd Week). MMWR Morb Mortal Wkly Rep. 2008 Jan 4;56(51-2):1361-9.

42.   CDC Healthcare Infection Control Practices Advisory Committee. Hand Hygiene in Healthcare Settings. http://www.cdc.gov/handhygiene/ Last revised 2007 May 8.

43.   CDC Select Agent Program Homepage. http://www.cdc.gov/od/sap/ Accessed 2007 Sep 7.

44.   Chang A, Tung RC, McGillis TS, Bergfeld WF, Taylor JS. Primary cutaneous coccidioidomycosis. J Am Acad Dermatol. 2003 Nov;49(5):944-9.

45.   Chasin BS, Elliott SP, Klotz SA. Medical errors arising from outsourcing laboratory and radiology services. Am J Med. 2007 Sep;120(9):819.e9-11.

46.   Chen X, Li W, Wang H. More tea for septic patients? Green tea may reduce endotoxin-induced release of high mobility group box 1 and other pro-inflammatory cytokines. Med Hypotheses. 2006;66(3):660-3. Epub 2005 Nov 2.

47.   Chew BP, Park JS. Carotenoid action on the immune response. J Nutr. 2004 Jan;134(1):257S-261S.

48.   Chiller TM, Galgiani JN, Stevens DA. Coccidioidomycosis. Infect Dis Clin North Am. 2003 Mar;17(1):41-57, viii.

49.   Chu JH, Feudtner C, Heydon K, Walsh TJ, Zaoutis TE. Hospitalizations for endemic mycoses: a population-based national study. Clin Infect Dis. 2006 Mar 15;42(6):822-5. Epub 2006 Feb 1.

50.   Chu JH, Zaoutis TE, Argon J, Feudtner C. National epidemiology of endemic fungal infections in children. Public Health and the Environment. The 132nd Annual Meeting (November 6-10, 2004) of the American Public Health Association (APHA). http://apha.confex.com/apha/132am/techprogram/paper_89147.htm Accessed 2006 Aug 02.

51.   Cleary JD, Rogers PD, Chapman SW. Variability in polyene content and cellular toxicity among deoxycholate amphotericin B formulations. Pharmacotherapy. 2003 May;23(5):572-8.

52.   Cohen IM, Galgiani JN, Potter D, Ogden DA. Coccidioidomycosis in renal replacement therapy. Arch Intern Med 1982 Mar;142(3):489-94.

53.   Cole GT. PhD, UTSA Department of Biology. Personal communication.

54.   Cole GT, Xue JM, Okeke CN, Tarcha EJ, Basrur V, Schaller RA, Herr RA, Yu JJ, Hung CY. A vaccine against coccidioidomycosis is justified and attainable. Med Mycol. 2004 Jun;42(3):189-216.

55.   Coleman MD. Phase I Enzyme Inhibition, p75-99 in Coleman MD. Human Drug Metabolism: An Introduction. Hoboken, NJ: John Wiley & Sons; 2005. 274p

56.   Collins BH, Horska A, Hotten PM, Riddoch C, Collins AR. Kiwifruit protects against oxidative DNA damage in human cells and in vitro. Nutr Cancer. 2001;39(1):148-53.

57.   Comrie AC. Climate factors influencing coccidioidomycosis seasonality and outbreaks. Environ Health Perspect. 2005 Jun;113(6):688-92.

58.   Cortez KJ, Walsh TJ, Bennett JE. Successful treatment of coccidioidal meningitis with voriconazole. Clin Infect Dis. 2003 Jun 15;36(12):1619-22. Epub 2003 Jun 09.

59.   County of Kern Department of Public Health. Coccidioidomycosis Cases Continue to Increase. Public Health Bulletin. 28 Nov 2002. http://www.co.kern.ca.us/health/pressr/coccy524.asp Accessed 12/30/2002.

60.   Crum NF, Ballon-Landa G. Coccidioidomycosis in pregnancy: case report and review of the literature. Am J Med. 2006 Nov;119(11):993.e11-7.

61.   Crum NF, Lamb C, Utz G, Amundson D, Wallace MR. Coccidioidomycosis outbreak among United States Navy SEALs training in a Coccidioides immitis-endemic area-Coalinga, California. J Infect Dis. 2002 Sep 15;186(6):865-8. Epub 2002 Aug 16.

62.   Crum NF, Lederman ER, Hale BR, Lim ML, Wallace MR. A cluster of disseminated coccidioidomycosis cases at a US military hospital. Mil Med. 2003 Jun;168(6):460-4.

63.   Crum NF, Lederman ER, Stafford CM, Parrish JS, Wallace MR. Coccidioidomycosis: A Descriptive Survey of a Reemerging Disease. Clinical Characteristics and Current Controversies. Medicine (Baltimore). 2004 May;83(3):149-175.

64.   Crum NF, Wallace MR. Laboratory Values Are Predictive of Disseminated Coccidioidomycosis. Inf Dis Clin Pract. 13(2):68-72, March 2005.

65.   Davis K. Public Relations Assistant for AABB, personal communication.

66.   Davis LE, Cook G, Costerton JW. Biofilm on ventriculo-peritoneal shunt tubing as a cause of treatment failure in coccidioidal meningitis. Emerg Infect Dis. 2002 Apr;8(4):376-9.

67.   Deaner RM, Einstein HE. Valley Fever. A primer for non-medical people. http://www.valleyfever.com/primer.htm Updated May 1999, Accessed 2006 May 9.

68.   Del Mundo NG, Garcia AL, Garcia K. Disseminated primary coccidioidomycosis during early third trimester of pregnancy results in rapid maternal death and neonatal demise despite aggressive treatment with amphotericin B. In Einstein, Hans E, Catanzaro, Antonio. (Eds) Coccidioidomycosis. Proceedings of the 5th International Conference on Coccidioidomycosis. Stanford University, 24-27 August, 1994. Washington DC: National Foundation for Infectious Diseases, 1996: p183-188.

69.   Deresinski SC. Coccidioidomycosis of bone and joints. In: Stevens DA. Coccidioidomycosis. A Text. New York, London: Plenum Medical Book Company, 1980: 195-211.

70.   Desai SA, Minai OA, Gordon SM, O'Neil B, Wiedemann HP, Arroliga AC. Coccidioidomycosis in non-endemic areas: a case series. Respir Med 2001 Apr;95(4):305-9.

71.   DiSalvo AF. Dimorphic Fungi. Microbiology and Immunology On-Line. http://pathmicro.med.sc.edu/mycology/mycology-6.htm Accessed 2006 Jul 8.

72.   Dixon DM. Coccidioides immitis as a Select Agent of bioterrorism. J Appl Microbiol. 2001 Oct;91(4):602-5.

73.   Dolan MJ, Lattuada CP, Melcher GP, Zellmer R, Allendoerfer R, Rinaldi MG. Coccidioides immitis presenting as a mycelial pathogen with empyema and hydropneumothorax. J Med Vet Mycol. 1992;30(3):249-55.

74.   Druginjurylaw.com - Law Offices of Thomas J. Lamb.   Remicade.
        http://www.druginjurylaw.com/Remicade-form.html Accessed 2004 Dec 2.

75.   Drutz DJ, Catanzaro A: Coccidioidomycosis. Part II. Am Rev Respir Dis.
        1978 Apr; 117(4): 727-71.

76.   Duthie SJ, Ma A, Ross MA, Collins AR. Antioxidant supplementation
        decreases oxidative DNA damage in human lymphocytes. Cancer Res. 1996
        Mar 15;56(6):1291-5.

77.   Edwards PQ, Palmer CE. Prevalence of sensitivity to coccidioidin, with
        special reference to specific and nonspecific reactions to coccidioidin and to
        histoplasmin. Dis Chest. 1957 Jan;31(1):35-60.

78.   Egeberg RO. Socioeconomic impact of coccidioidomycosis. In: Einstein
        HE, Catanzaro A, eds. Coccidioidomycosis. Proceedings of the 4th
        International Conference on Coccidioidomycosis. Washington, DC.
        National Foundation for Infectious Diseases; 1985: 27-33.

79.   Einstein HE, Johnson RH. Coccidioidomycosis: new aspects of
        epidemiology and therapy. Clin Infect Dis 1993;16:349-56.

80.   Ellis D. Amphotericin B: spectrum and resistance. J Antimicrob
        Chemother. 2002 Feb;49 Suppl 1:7-10.

81.   Engelthaler D quoted in Thorson S. Valley Fever Cases Rise Sharply. East
        Valley Tribune. 2006 Apr 4.

82.   FDA Center for Devices and Radiological Health. FDA Public Health
        Notification: Reducing Radiation Risk from Computed Tomography for
        Pediatric and Small Adult Patients.
        http://www.fda.gov/cdrh/safety/110201-ct.html 2001 Nov 2. Accessed
        2008 Jan 9.

83.   FDA Center for Drug Evaluation and Research. Information for Healthcare
        Professionals Gadolinium-Based Contrast Agents for Magnetic Resonance
        Imaging.
        http://www.fda.gov/CDER/drug/InfoSheets/HCP/gcca_200705.htm Last
        updated 2007 May 23.

84.   FDA Center for Drug Evaluation and Research. Posaconazole Patient
        Information Sheet.
        http://www.fda.gov/cder/drug/InfoSheets/patient/posaconazolePIS.htm
        2007 Jan 30. Accessed 2007 May 10.

85.   FDA Center for Drug Evaluation and Research. The Safety of Sporanox
        Capsules and Lamisil Tablets for the Treatment of Onychomycosis. FDA
        Public Health Advisory.
        http://www.fda.gov/CDER/drug/advisory/sporanox-lamisil/advisory.htm
        Last Updated: 2001 May 09.

86.   Fiese MJ. Epidemiology of coccidioidomycosis. In: Fiese MJ.
        Coccidioidomycosis. Springfield, Charles C. Thomas, 1958. 77-91.

87.   Fiese MJ. The History of Coccidioidomycosis. In: Fiese MJ.
        Coccidioidomycosis. Springfield, Charles C. Thomas, 1958. 10-22.

88.   Fiese MJ. Therapy of coccidioidomycosis. In Ferguson MS, ed. Proceedings of Symposium on Coccidioidomycosis. Atlanta, Public Health Service Publication No. 575, 1957.

89.   Fiese MJ. Variations in susceptibility to coccidioidal infection. In: Fiese MJ. Coccidioidomycosis. Springfield, Charles C. Thomas, 1958. 101-103.

90.   Fiese MJ. Treatment of Coccidioidomycosis. In Fiese MJ. Coccidioidomycosis. Springfield, Charles C. Thomas, 1958: 174-186.

91.   Fish DG, Ampel NM, Galgiani JN, Dols CL, Kelly PC, Johnson CH, Pappagianis D, Edwards JE, Wasserman RB, Clark RJ, et al. Coccidioidomycosis during human immunodeficiency virus infection. A review of 77 patients. Medicine (Baltimore). 1990 Nov;69(6):384-91.

92.   Fisher MC, Koenig GL, White TJ, Taylor JW. Molecular and phenotypic description of Coccidioides posadasii sp. nov., previously recognized as the non-California population of Coccidioides immitis. Mycologia. 2002; 94: 73-84.

93.   Fortun J, Martin-Davila P, Moreno S, Barcena R, De Vicente E, Honrubia A, Garcia M, Nuno J, Candela A, Uriarte M, Pintado V. Prevention of invasive fungal infections in liver transplant recipients: the role of prophylaxis with lipid formulations of amphotericin B in high-risk patients. J Antimicrob Chemother. 2003 Nov;52(5):813-9. Epub 2003 Oct 16.

94.   Fromtling RA, Shadomy HJ. An overview of macrophage-fungal interactions. Mycopathologia 1986 Feb;93(2):77-93.

95.   Galgiani JN. Coccidioidomycosis: A Regional Disease of National Importance. Ann Int Med 1999 Vol 130 No 4 (part 1) p293-300.

96.   Galgiani JN. Personal communication.

97.   Galgiani JN. Valley Fever Center for Excellence (VFCE) Annual Report 2001-2002. Tucson, Arizona: University of Arizona 2002.

98.   Galgiani JN, Ampel NM, Blair JE, Catanzaro A, Johnson RH, Stevens DA, Williams PL. IDSA Guidelines. Coccidioidomycosis. Clin Inf Dis. 2005;41:1217-1223.

99.   Galgiani JN, Ampel NM, Catanzaro A, Johnson RH, Stevens DA, Williams PL. Practice guideline for the treatment of coccidioidomycosis. Infectious Diseases Society of America. Clin Infect Dis. 2000 Apr;30(4):658-61. Epub 2000 Apr 20.

100.   Galgiani JN, Brauer RJ. Valley Fever Center for Excellence Annual Report 2002-2003. Tucson, Arizona: University of Arizona 2003.

101.   Galgiani JN, Catanzaro A, Cloud GA, Higgs J, Friedman BA, Larsen RA, Graybill JR, NIAID-Mycoses Study Group. Fluconazole therapy for coccidioidal meningitis. Ann Intern Med. 1993 Jul 1;119(1):28-35.

102.   Galgiani JN, Catanzaro A, Cloud GA, Johnson RH, Williams PL, Mirels LF, Nassar F, Lutz JE, Stevens DA, Sharkey PK, Singh VR, Larsen RA, Delgado KL, Flanigan C, Rinaldi MG, NIAID-Mycoses Study Group. Comparison of oral fluconazole and itraconazole for progressive, nonmeningeal

coccidioidomycosis. A randomized, double-blind trial. Ann Intern Med. 2000 Nov 7;133(9):676-86.

103.   Gelhlbach SH, Hamilton JD, Connant NF. Coccidioidomycosis-an occupational disease in cotton mill workers. Arch Intern Med 1973;131:254-5.

104.   Gerberding JL quoted in CDC. Press Release: Hand Hygiene in Healthcare Settings. Accessible online at http://www.cdc.gov/handhygiene/pressrelease.htm 2002 Oct 25.

105.   Gibbs BT, Neff RT. A 22-year-old Army private with chest pain and weight loss. Mil Med. 2004 Feb;169(2):157-60.

106.   Gifford MA, Buss WC, Douds RJ. Data on coccidioides fungus infection. Kern County, 1901-1936. In: Annual Report of the Kern County Department of Public Health, 1936-37, p39-54.

107.   Gokhale S, Logrono R, Walser EM. Solitary pulmonary nodule found incidentally in a smoker at Galveston, Texas. Diagn Cytopathol. 2003 Feb;28(2):110-1.

108.   Gonzalez GM, Tijerina R, Najvar LK, Bocanegra R, Luther M, Rinaldi MG, Graybill JR. Correlation between antifungal susceptibilities of Coccidioides immitis in vitro and antifungal treatment with caspofungin in a mouse model. Antimicrob Agents Chemother. 2001 Jun;45(6):1854-9.

109.   Gonzalez GM, Tijerina R, Najvar LK, Bocanegra R, Rinaldi M, Loebenberg D, Graybill JR. In vitro and in vivo activities of posaconazole against Coccidioides immitis. Antimicrob Agents Chemother. 2002 May;46(5):1352-6.

110.   Goodman DH. Systemic fungal infection complications in asthmatic patients treated with steroids. Ann Allergy. 1973 Apr;31(4):205-8.

111.   Graybill JR. Future directions of antifungal chemotherapy. Clin Infect Dis. 1992 Mar;14 Suppl 1:S170-81.

112.   Graybill JR, Revankar SG, Patterson TF. Antifungal agents and antifungal susceptibility testing. In: Collier L, Balows A, Sussman M, Ajello L, Hay RJ, eds. 9th ed. Topley and Wilson's microbiology and microbial infections, Vol. 4, Medical Mycology. London: Arnold; New York: Oxford University Press, 1998: 163-175.

113.   Hagman HM, Madnick EG, D'Agostino AN, Williams PL, Shatsky S, Mirels LF, Tucker RM, Rinaldi MG, Stevens DA, Bryant RE. Hyphal forms in the central nervous system of patients with coccidioidomycosis. Clin Infect Dis 2000 Feb;30(2):349-53.

114.   Halpern AA, Rinsky LA, Fountain S, Nagel DA. Coccidioidomycosis of the spine: unusual roentgenographic presentation. Clin Orthop 1979 May;(140):78-9.

115.   Hardy Diagnostics. Premier Coccidioides. http://www.hardydiagnostics.com/catalog2/hugo/Premier-Coccidioides.htm Accessed 2008 Feb 10.

116.   HCUP Databases. Arizona, State Inpatient Databases (SID), Healthcare Cost and Utilization Project (HCUP), Agency for Healthcare Research and Quality. http://hcupnet.ahrq.gov/ Accessed 2008 Jan 17.

117.   Hector RF, Davidson AP, Johnson SM. Comparison of susceptibility of fungal isolates to lufenuron and nikkomycin Z alone or in combination with itraconazole. Am J Vet Res. 2005 Jun;66(6):1090-3.

118.   Hector RF, Rutherford GW. The public health need and present status of a vaccine for the prevention of coccidioidomycosis. Ann N Y Acad Sci. 2007 Sep;1111:259-68. Epub 2007 Mar 7.

119.   Hector RF, Zimmer BL, Pappagianis D. Evaluation of nikkomycins X and Z in murine models of coccidioidomycosis, histoplasmosis, and blastomycosis. Chemother. 1990 Apr;34(4):587-93.

120.   HHS, CDC, NIH. Biosafety in Microbiological and Biomedical Laboratories (BMBL) 5th Edition. U.S. Department of Health and Human Services, Centers for Disease Control and Prevention, and National Institutes of Health. Fifth Edition, Feb 2007. US Government Printing Office. Washington: 2007. Accessible online at http://www.cdc.gov/od/ohs/biosfty/bmbl5/bmbl5toc.htm

121.   Hogan LH, Klein BS, Levitz SM. Virulence Factors of Medically Important Fungi. Clin Microbiol Rev. 1996 Oct;9(4): 469-488.

122.   Holley K, Muldoon M, Tasker S. Coccidioides immitis osteomyelitis: a case series review. Orthopedics 2002 Aug;25(8):827-31, 831-2.

123.   Hooper JE, Lu Q, Pepkowitz SH. Disseminated coccidioidomycosis in pregnancy. Arch Pathol Lab Med. 2007 Apr;131(4):652-5.

124.   Horton JW. Free radicals and lipid peroxidation mediated injury in burn trauma: the role of antioxidant therapy. Toxicology. 2003 Jul 15;189(1-2):75-88.

125.   Howell, Michael. http://www.arachnoiditis.net/ Accessed 2004 June 15.

126.   Hsue G, Napier JT, Prince RA, Chi J, Hospenthal DR. Treatment of meningeal coccidioidomycosis with caspofungin. J Antimicrob Chemother. 2004 Jul;54(1):292-4.

127.   Hung CY, Xue J, Cole GT. Virulence mechanisms of coccidioides. Ann N Y Acad Sci. 2007 Oct;1111:225-35. Epub 2007 May 18.

128.   Huntington RW. Morphology and racial distribution of fatal coccidioidomycosis. JAMA 169:115-119, 1959.

129.   Huntington RW. Pathology of coccidioidomycosis. In: Stevens DA. Coccidioidomycosis. A Text. New York, London: Plenum Medical Book Company, 1980: 113-132.

130.   Huppert M. Coccidioides immitis: structure and function or know thy adversary. In: Einstein HE, Catanzaro A, eds. Coccidioidomycosis. Proceedings of the 4th International Conference on Coccidioidomycosis. Washington, DC. National Foundation for Infectious Diseases; 1985: 77-87.

131.   Huppert M, Sun SH. Mycological Diagnosis of Coccidioidomycosis. In: Stevens DA. ed. Coccidioidomycosis, a text. New York: Plenum Medical Book Company, 1980: 47-61.

132.   Huppert M, Sun SH, Gleason-Jordon I, Vukovich KR. Lung weight parallels disease severity in experimental coccidioidomycosis. Infect Immun. 1976 Dec;14(6):1356-68.

133.   Hussein G, Sankawa U, Goto H, Matsumoto K, Watanabe H. Astaxanthin, a carotenoid with potential in human health and nutrition. J Nat Prod. 2006 Mar;69(3):443-9.

134.   Iger M, Coppola AJ. Review of 135 cases of bone and joint coccidioidomycosis. In: Einstein HE, Catanzaro A, eds. Coccidioidomycosis. Proceedings of the 4th International Conference on Coccidioidomycosis. Washington, DC. National Foundation for Infectious Diseases; 1985: 379-389.

135.   Immuno-Mycologics. Coccidioides Latex Agglutination/Immunodiffusion combination Kit - 40 Tests. Package Insert. http://www.immy.com/pkgins/CI1001.pdf Accessed 2006 May 30.

136.   Immuno-Mycologics. Omega Coccidioides Antibody EIA REF CAB102. Package Insert. http://www.immy.com/pkgins/CI1001.pdf Accessed 2006 May 30.

137.   Injury Lawyer Network. Sporanox Anti-Fungal Treatment. http://www.injury-lawyer-network.com/sporanox.htm Accessed 2005 Feb 22.

138.   Jacobs PH. Cutaneous Coccidioidomycosis. In: Stevens DA. Coccidioidomycosis. A Text. New York, London: Plenum Medical Book Company, 1980: 213-224.

139.   Johnson LR, Herrgesell EJ, Davidson AP, Pappagianis D. Clinical, clinicopathologic, and radiographic findings in dogs with coccidioidomycosis: 24 cases (1995-2000). J Am Vet Med Assoc. 2003 Feb 15;222(4):461-6.

140.   Johnson RH, Brown JF, Holeman CW, Helvie SJ, Einstein HE. Coccidioidal meningitis: a 25-year experience with 194 patients. In: Einstein HE, Catanzaro A, eds. Coccidioidomycosis. Proceedings of the 4th International Conference on Coccidioidomycosis. Washington, DC. National Foundation for Infectious Diseases; 1985: 411-421.

141.   Johnson RH, Einstein HE. Amphotericin B and coccidioidomycosis. Ann N Y Acad Sci. 2007 Sep;1111:434-41. Epub 2007 May 18.

142.   Johnson RH, Einstein HE. Forty-five years of disseminated coccidioidomycosis. In: Proceedings of the Forty-Sixth Annual Coccidioidomycosis Study Group Meeting. March 31, 2001. The University of Arizona. April 6, 2002. Davis, California. VFCE. http://www.vfce.arizona.edu/csg/csg45.htm accessed 2005 Jun 13.

143.   Johnson WM. Coccidioidomycosis mortality in Arizona. In: Ajello L, editor. Coccidioidomycosis: Current clinical and diagnostic status. Miami: Symposia Specialists; 1977: 33-44.

144.   Jones FL Jr, Spivey CG Jr. Spread of pulmonary coccidioidomycosis associated with steroid therapy. Report of a case with a lupus-like reaction to antituberculosis chemotherapy. J Lancet. 1966 May;86(5):226-30.

145.   Jones JL, Fleming PL, Ciesielski CA et al.: Coccidioidomycosis among persons with AIDS in the United States. J Infect Dis. 171:961-6, 1995.

146.   Kanal E, Broome DR, Martin DR, Thomsen HS. Response to the FDA's May 23, 2007, Nephrogenic Systemic Fibrosis Update. Radiology. 2008 Jan;246(1):11-4.

147.   Kaufman L, Sekhon AS, Moledina N, Jalbert M, Pappagianis D. Comparative evaluation of commercial Premier EIA and microimmunodiffusion and complement fixation tests for Coccidioides immitis antibodies. J Clin Microbiol. 1995 Mar;33(3):618-9.

148.   Kelly PC. Coccidioidal meningitis. In: Einstein HE, Catanzaro A, eds. Coccidioidomycosis. Proceedings of the 5th International Conference on Coccidioidomycosis. Stanford University, 24-27 August, 1994. Washington, DC. National Foundation for Infectious Diseases; 1996: 373-384.

149.   Kim J, Sporer R, Jean B, Peck R. Pediatric coccidioidomycosis meningitis with hydrocephalus and pancreatitis. In Einstein, Hans E, Catanzaro, Antonio. (Eds) Coccidioidomycosis. Proceedings of the 5th International Conference on Coccidioidomycosis. Stanford University, 24-27 August, 1994. Washington DC: National Foundation for Infectious Diseases, 1996: p188-193.

150.   Kirkland TN, Fierer J. Coccidioidomycosis: a reemerging infectious disease. Emerg Infect Dis. 1996 Jul-Sep;2(3):192-9.

151.   Knight JA. Review: Free radicals, antioxidants, and the immune system. Ann Clin Lab Sci. 2000 Apr;30(2):145-58.

152.   Kolivras KN, Comrie AC. Modeling valley fever (coccidioidomycosis) incidence on the basis of climate conditions. Int J Biometeorol. 2003 Mar;47(2):87-101.

153.   Kolivras KN, Johnson PS, Comrie AC, Yool SR. Environmental Variability and Coccidioidomycosis (Valley Fever). 2001 Aerobiologia 17, 31-42.

154.   Kotwani RN, Bodhe PV, Kirodian BG, Mehta KP, Ali US, Kshirsagar NA. Indian Pediatr. Treatment of neonatal candidiasis with liposomal amphotericin B(L-AMP-LRC-1): phase II study. 2003 Jun;40(6):545-50.

155.   Krohne SG. Canine systemic fungal infections. Vet Clin North Am Small Anim Pract 2000 Sep;30(5):1063-90.

156.   Laboratory Alliance of Central New York, LLC. Coccidioides Antibodies, IgG & IgM by ELISA. http://www.laboratoryalliance.com/dirofser.cfm?action=searchdetails&order_id=1093 Accessed 2008 Feb 10.

157.   Laniado-Laborín R. Cost-benefit analysis of treating acute coccidioidal pneumonia with azole drugs. In: Proceedings of the Forty-Fifth Annual Coccidioidomycosis Study Group Meeting. March 31, 2001. The University of Arizona. Tucson, Arizona. http://www.vfce.arizona.edu/csg/csg45.htm Accessed 6/13/05.

158.   Lavetter A. Coccidioidomycosis in pediatrics. In: Stevens DA. Coccidioidomycosis. A Text. New York, London: Plenum Medical Book Company, 1980: 245-248.

159.   Lawrence MA, Ginsberg D, Stein JP, Kanel G, Skinner DG. Coccidioidomycosis prostatitis associated with prostate cancer. BJU Int. 1999 Aug;84(3):372-3.

160.   Leake JA, Mosley DG, England B, Graham JV, Plikaytis BD, Ampel NM, Perkins BA, Hajjeh RA. Risk factors for acute symptomatic coccidioidomycosis among elderly persons in Arizona, 1996-1997. J Infect Dis. 2000 Apr;181(4):1435-40. Epub 2000 Apr 07.

161.   Leonard B. Stress, depression and the activation of the immune system. World J Biol Psychiatry 2000 Jan;1(1):17-25.

162.   Leontic EA. Respiratory disease in pregnancy. Med Clin North Am. 1977 Jan;61(1):111-28.

163.   Lewicky YM, Roberto RF, Curtin SL. The unique complications of coccidioidomycosis of the spine: a detailed time line of disease progression and suppression. Spine. 2004 Oct 1;29(19):E435-41.

164.   Lin ZB. Cellular and molecular mechanisms of immuno-modulation by Ganoderma lucidum. J Pharmacol Sci. 2005 Oct;99(2):144-53.

165.   Linsangan LC, Ross LA. Coccidioides immitis infection of the neonate: two routes of infection. Pediatr Infect Dis J. 1999 Feb;18(2):171-3.

166.   Los Angeles County. Tables of Notifiable Diseases 2006. http://www.lapublichealth.org/acd/docs/Tablesnotifynew06%5B1%5D.pdf Updated 2007 Oct 29, accessed 2007 Nov 4.

167.   Los Angeles County Department of Public Health. Questions and Answers About Valley Fever (coccidioidomycosis or "cocci"). http://www.lapublichealth.org/acd/docs/Health%20Education/CocciFinal.pdf Accessed 2008 Apr 15.

168.   Louie L, Ng S, Hajjeh R, Johnson R, Vugia D, Werner SB, Talbot R, Klitz W. Influence of host genetics on the severity of coccidioidomycosis. Emerg Infect Dis. 1999 Sep-Oct;5(5):672-80.

169.   Mandel S, Amit T, Reznichenko L, Weinreb O, Youdim MB. Green tea catechins as brain-permeable, natural iron chelators-antioxidants for the treatment of neurodegenerative disorders. Mol Nutr Food Res. 2006 Feb;50(2):229-34

170.   Marmor D. "Fungus among us" and Workmen's Compensation. Med Trial Tech Q. 1976 Spring;22(4):385-402.

171.   McBride J. High-ORAC Foods May Slow Aging. USDA Agricultural Research Service. 1999 Feb 8. http://www.ars.usda.gov/is/pr/1999/990208.htm Accessed 2007 Jan 28.

172.   McCarthy K. FY09 Budget Request. Representative Kevin McCarthy's letter to Office of Management and Budget Director Jim Nussle was co-signed by the following U.S. Representatives: Devin Nunes, Ken Calvert, Jim Costa, George Radanovich, Darrell Issa, Rick Renzi, Raul Grijalva, Stevan Pearce,

and Jon C. Porter. 2007 Dec 20. Received from the Valley Fever Americas Foundation on 2008 Jan 9.

173.   McCarthy KL, Playford EG, Looke DF, Whitby M. Severe photosensitivity causing multifocal squamous cell carcinomas secondary to prolonged voriconazole therapy. Clin Infect Dis. 2007 Mar 1;44(5):e55-6.

174.   McCoy MJ, Ellenberg JF, Killam AP. Coccidioidomycosis complicating pregnancy. Am J Obstet Gynecol 1980;137:739-40.

175.   MDA. Coccidioidomycosis. MDA Internet. http://www.mdainternet.com/topics_c/coccidioidomycosis.htm Accessed 2002 Sept 05.

176.   Medline Plus Drug Information. http://www.nlm.nih.gov/medlineplus/druginformation.html Accessed 2007 Feb 19.

177.   Merck. Coccidioidomycosis. The Merck Manual of Diagnosis and Therapy. Sec. 13, Ch. 158, Systemic Fungal Diseases. http://www.merck.com/mrkshared/mmanual/section13/chapter158/158c.jsp Accessed 2004 July 14.

178.   Merchant M, Romero AO, Libke RD, Joseph J. Pleural effusion in hospitalized patients with Coccidioidomycosis. Respir Med. 2007 Dec 28 [Epub ahead of print]

179.   Miller J, Engelberg S, Broad WJ. Germs: biological weapons and America's secret war. New York: Simon & Schuster, 2001.

180.   Miller MB, Hendren R, Gilligan PH. Posttransplantation disseminated coccidioidomycosis acquired from donor lungs. J Clin Microbiol. 2004 May;42(5):2347-9.

181.   Minutes of the Arizona State Senate Committee on Health. Phoenix, AZ 4 Feb 2002. http://www.azleg.state.az.us/FormatDocument.asp?inDoc=/legtext/46leg/1R/comm_min/Senate/0213+HEA%2EDOC.htm Accessed 8/01/2003.

182.   MiraVista Diagnostics. Case Studies: Therapy for coccidioidomycosis. http://www.miravistalabs.com/refLibrary_caseStudies_pageCocci.php Accessed 2006 Apr 23.

183.   Mirbod-Donovan F, Schaller R, Hung CY, Xue J, Reichard U, Cole GT. Urease produced by Coccidioides posadasii contributes to the virulence of this respiratory pathogen. Infect Immun. 2006 Jan;74(1):504-15.

184.   Morino E, Naka G, Izumi S, Yoshizawa A, Kawana A, Toyota E, Kobayashi N, Kudo K. Case of cavitary coccidioidomycosis with fungus balls in the apices of both lungs. Nihon Kokyuki Gakkai Zasshi. 2006 Oct;44(10):711-5. Abstract translated at Pubmed.

185.   Nagda NL, Fortmann MD, Koontz MD, Baker SR, Ginevan ME. Airliner Cabin Environment: Contaminant Measurements, Health Risks, and Mitigation Options. DOT-P-15–89–5. NTIS/PB91–159384. Prepared by GEOMET Technologies, Germantown, MD, for the U.S. Department of Transportation, Washington DC. 1989.

186.   Natureworks LLC.   Free radicals, antioxidants, the immune system.
        http://www.immunedisorders.homestead.com/radicals.html Accessed 2007
        Apr 4.

187.   Nicas M, Hubbard A.   A risk analysis for airborne pathogens with low
        infectious doses: application to respirator selection against Coccidioides
        immitis spores. Risk Anal 2002 Dec;22(6):1153-63.

188.   NINDS. NINDS Arachnoiditis Information Page.   National Institute of
        Neurological Disorders and Stroke.
        http://www.ninds.nih.gov/disorders/arachnoiditis/arachnoiditis.htm
        Accessed 2006 Dec 11.

189.   Ogiso A, Ito M, Koyama M, Yamaoka H, Hotchi M, McGinnis MR. 1997.
        Pulmonary coccidioidomycosis in Japan: case report and review. Clin. Infect.
        Dis. 25:1260-1261.

190.   Oldfield EC 3rd, Bone WD, Martin CR, Gray GC, Olson P, Schillaci RF.
        Prediction of relapse after treatment of coccidioidomycosis. Clin Infect Dis.
        1997 Nov;25(5):1205-10.

191.   O'Neil J. Hazards: All Dressed Up, Carrying Germs. The New York Times.
        Published 2004 May 25.
        http://www.nytimes.com/2004/05/25/health/25haza.html Accessed 17
        Jan 2007.

192.   Palazzetti S, Rousseau AS, Richard MJ, Favier A, Margaritis I. Antioxidant
        supplementation preserves antioxidant response in physical training and low
        antioxidant intake. Br J Nutr. 2004 Jan;91(1):91-100.

193.   Papadopoulos KI, Castor B, Klingspor L, Dejmek A, Loren I, Bramnert M.
        Bilateral isolated adrenal coccidioidomycosis.   J Intern Med. 1996
        Mar;239(3):275-8.

194.   Pappagianis D. Clinical presentation of Infectious Entities. In: Einstein HE,
        Catanzaro A, eds. Coccidioidomycosis. Proceedings of the 5th International
        Conference on Coccidioidomycosis.   Stanford University, 24-27 August,
        1994. Washington, DC. National Foundation for Infectious Diseases; 1996:
        9-11.

195.   Pappagianis D. Coccidioidomycosis (San Joaquin or Valley Fever). In:
        DiSalvo AF, ed. Occupational Mycoses. Philadelphia: Lea & Febiger; 1983:
        13-28.

196.   Park DW, Sohn JW, Cheong HJ, Kim WJ, Kim MJ, Kim JH, Shin C.
        Combination therapy of disseminated coccidioidomycosis with caspofungin
        and fluconazole. BMC Infect Dis. 2006 Feb 15;6:26.

197.   Perricone N. Dr. Perricone's 7 secrets to beauty, health, and longevity: the
        miracle of cellular rejuvenation. New York : Ballantine Books, c2006. 333p.

198.   Perricone N. The Perricone promise: look younger, live longer in three easy
        steps. New York: Warner Books, c2004. 307p.

199.   Perricone N. The Perricone weight-loss diet: a simple 3-part plan to lose the
        fat, the wrinkles, and the years. New York: Ballantine Books, c2005. 300p.

200.   Peter JB. Coccidioides immitis. Specialty Laboratories. Use &
        Interpretation of Laboratory Tests Books.
        http://www.specialtylabs.com/books/display.asp?id=321 Accessed 2006
        August 30.

201.   Pitisuttithum P, Negroni R, Graybill JR, Bustamante B, Pappas P, Chapman
        S, Hare RS, Hardalo CJ. Activity of posaconazole in the treatment of central
        nervous system fungal infections. J Antimicrob Chemother. 2005
        Oct;56(4):745-55.

202.   Pollage CR, et al. Revisiting the sensitivity of serologic testing in culture
        positive coccidioidomycosis. Presented at the 106th Annual Meeting of the
        American Society of Microbiology. Orlando, FL. 2006. Cited in: Saubolle
        MA. Laboratory aspects in the diagnosis of coccidioidomycosis. Ann N Y
        Acad Sci. 2007 Sep;1111:301-14. Epub 2007 Mar 15.

203.   Pont A, Williams PL, Azhar S, Reitz RE, Bochra C, Smith ER, Stevens DA.
        Ketoconazole blocks testosterone synthesis. Arch Intern Med. 1982
        Nov;142(12):2137-40.

204.   Rao S, Biddle M, Balchum OJ, Robinson JL. Focal endemic
        coccidioidomycosis in Los Angeles County. Am Rev Respir Dis 1972
        Mar;105(3):410-6

205.   Reardon J. Valley Fever: It's in the air. KVOA 4 News. Tuscon, AZ. 2004
        September 24 at 5:21pm MST.
        http://kvoa.com/Global/story.asp?S=2347067 Accessed online 2007 Dec
        3.

206.   Reed RE, Ingram KA, Reggiardo C, Shupe MR. Coccidioidomycosis in
        domestic and wild animals. In Einstein, Hans E, Catanzaro, Antonio. (Eds)
        Coccidioidomycosis. Proceedings of the 5th International Conference on
        Coccidioidomycosis. Stanford University, 24-27 August, 1994. Washington
        DC: National Foundation for Infectious Diseases, 1996: 146-154.

207.   Ricci~Leopold Consumer Justice Attorneys. Nash v. Centocor, Inc.,
        Johnson & Johnson, Orth-McNeil Pharmaceutical, Inc., John Doe
        Manufacturers A-Z, and John Doe Distributors A-Z.
        http://www.riccilegal.com/CM/News/Complaint - Centocor.doc Accessed
        2004 Dec 2.

208.   Roberts PL, Lisciandro RC. A community epidemic of coccidioidomycosis.
        Am Rev Respir Dis. 1967 Oct;96(4):766-72.

209.   Romeo JH, Rice LB, McQuarrie IG. Hydrocephalus in coccidioidal
        meningitis: case report and review of the literature. Neurosurgery 2000
        Sep;47(3):773-7.

210.   Rosenstein NE, Emery KW, Werner SB, Kao A, Johnson R, Rogers D,
        Vugia D, Reingold A, Talbot R, Plikaytis BD, Perkins BA, Hajjeh RA. Risk
        factors for severe pulmonary and disseminated coccidioidomycosis: Kern
        County, California, 1995-1996. Clin Infect Dis. 2001 Mar 1;32(5):708-15.
        Epub 2001 Feb 28.

211.   Rothman PE, Graw RG Jr, Harris JC Jr, Onslow JM. Coccidiodomycosis--
        possible fomite transmission. A review and report of a case. Am J Dis Child.
        1969 Nov;118(5):792-801.

212.   Salkin D. Clinical examples of reinfection in coccidioidomycosis. Am Rev
        Respir Dis. 1967 Apr;95(4):603-11.

213.   Saiontz, Kirk and Miles, P.A.   Gadolinium Side Effects: MRI Contrast
        Dangers.   http://www.youhavealawyer.com/gadolinium/gadolinium-side-
        effects.html Accessed 2007 Nov 20.

214.   Salkin D. Clinical examples of reinfection in coccidioidomycosis. Ajello L,
        ed.   Coccidioidomycosis.   Papers from the second symposium on
        coccidioidomycosis. Tucson: University of Arizona Press, 1967: 11-18.

215.   Saubolle MA. Laboratory aspects in the diagnosis of coccidioidomycosis.
        Ann N Y Acad Sci. 2007 Sep;1111:301-14. Epub 2007 Mar 15.

216.   Saubolle MA. Life Cycle and epidemiology of Coccidioides immitis. In:
        Einstein HE, Catanzaro A, eds. Coccidioidomycosis. Proceedings of the 5th
        International Conference on Coccidioidomycosis. Stanford University, 24-27
        August, 1994. Washington, DC. National Foundation for Infectious
        Diseases; 1996: 1-8.

217.   Saubolle MA, McKellar PP, Sussland D.   Epidemiologic, clinical, and
        diagnostic aspects of coccidioidomycosis.   J Clin Microbiol. 2007
        Jan;45(1):26-30.

218.   Schmelzer LL, Tabershaw IR.   Exposure factors in occupational
        coccidioidomycosis. Am J. Public Health 58:107-113, Jan 1968.

219.   Schmidt RT, Howard DH. Possibility of C. immitis infection of museum
        personnel. Public Health Rep, 1968, 83, 882. Cited in: Drutz DJ, Catanzaro
        A: Coccidioidomycosis. Part I. Am Rev Respir Dis 1978 Mar; 117(3): 559-85.

220.   Schmidt H, Martindale R. The gastrointestinal tract in critical illness:
        nutritional implications. Curr Opin Clin Nutr Metab Care. 2003 Sep;6(5):587-
        91.

221.   Schwarz J. What's new in mycotic bone and joint diseases? Pathol Res Pract
        1984 Jul;178(6):617-34.

222.   Semelka RC, Armao DM, Elias J Jr, Huda W. Imaging strategies to reduce
        the risk of radiation in CT studies, including selective substitution with MRI.
        J Magn Reson Imaging. 2007 May;25(5):900-9.

223.   Shibli M, Ghassibi J, Hajal R, O'Sullivan M.   Adjunctive corticosteroids
        therapy in acute respiratory distress syndrome owing to disseminated
        coccidioidomycosis. Crit Care Med. 2002 Aug;30(8):1896-8.

224.   Shubitz LF. Comparative Aspects of Coccidioidomycosis in Animals and
        Humans. Ann N Y Acad Sci. 2007 Mar 1;1111:396-.403

225.   Shubitz LF. Do dogs get valley fever?
        http://vfce.arl.arizona.edu/vek9vf.htm Accessed 2004 Mar 13.

226.   Shubitz LF. Incidence of Infection Study Results.
        http://www.vfce.arizona.edu/VFID-results.htm Accessed 2007 Oct 16.

227.   Shubitz LF, Peng T, Perrill R, Simons J, Orsborn K, Galgiani JN. Protection
        of mice against Coccidioides immitis intranasal infection by vaccination with
        recombinant antigen 2/PRA. Infect Immun. 2002 Jun;70(6):3287-9.

228. Singh SS, Caldwell JW, Johnson RH, Einstein HE, Williams PL. Safety and tolerance of high dose fluconazole in disseminated coccidioidomycosis. In Einstein HE, Catanzaro A, eds. Coccidioidomycosis. Proceedings of the 5th International Conference on Coccidioidomycosis. Stanford University, 24-27 August, 1994. Washington, DC. National Foundation for Infectious Diseases; 1996: P285-301.

229. Singh VR, Smith DK, Lawerence J, Kelly PC, Thomas AR, Spitz B, Sarosi GA. Coccidioidomycosis in patients infected with human immunodeficiency virus: review of 91 cases at a single institution. Clin Infect Dis. 1996 Sep;23(3):563-8.

230. Smale LE, Waechter KG. Dissemination of coccidioidomycosis in pregnancy. Am J Obstet Gynecol. 1970 Jun 1;107(3):356-61.

231. Smilack JD, Argueta R. Coccidioidal infection of the thyroid. Arch Intern Med 1998 Jan 12;158(1):89-92.

232. Smith CE. Personal communication to authors in: Smith DT, Harrell ER, Jr. Fatal coccidioidomycosis. A case of a laboratory infection. Am. Rev. Tuberc 1948 Jan; 57:368-374.

233. Smith CE, Saito MT, Simons SA. Pattern of 39,500 serologic tests in coccidioidomycosis. JAMA. 1956;160:546-552.

234. Snyder CH. Coccidioidal meningitis presenting as memory loss. J Am Acad Nurse Pract. 2005 May;17(5):181-6.

235. Solomon S quoted in: CDC. Press Release: Hand Hygiene in Healthcare Settings. Accessible online at http://www.cdc.gov/handhygiene/pressrelease.htm 2002 Oct 25.

236. Specialty Laboratories. #2526: Coccidioides Total Antibodies. Specialty Laboratories Test Menu. http://www.specialtylabs.com/tests/details.asp?id=2526 Accessed 2007 Dec 03.

237. Spinello IM, Johnson RH, Baqi S. Coccidioidomycosis and pregnancy: a review. Ann N Y Acad Sci. 2007 Sep;1111:358-64. Epub 2007 Mar 15.

238. Stack S. Valley Fever - The Arizona Disease. Arizona Adopt a Greyhound, Inc. http://www.arizonaadoptagreyhound.org/valley_fever.html Accessed 2005 Feb 28.

239. Standaert SM, Schaffner W, Galgiani JN, Pinner RW, Kaufman L, Durry E, Hutcheson RH. Coccidioidomycosis among visitors to a Coccidioides immitis-endemic area: an outbreak in a military reserve unit. J Infect Dis 1995 Jun;171(6):1672-5.

240. Stevens DA. Current concepts: Coccidioidomycosis. N Engl J Med. 1995 Apr 20;332(16):1077-82.

241. Stevens DA. Diagnosis of fungal infections: current status. J Antimicrob Chemother. 2002 Feb;49 Suppl 1:11-9.

242. Stevens DA. Immunology of coccidioidomycosis. In: Stevens DA. Coccidioidomycosis. A Text. New York, London: Plenum Medical Book Company, 1980: 87-95.

243.   Stevens DA. Overview of amphotericin B colloidal dispersion (amphocil). J Infect. 1994 May;28 Suppl 1:45-9.

244.   Sunenshine RH. CDC and ADHS, Personal Communication.

245.   Swatek FE. Epidemiology of coccidioidomycosis. In: Al-Doory, Y (ed). The Epidemiology of Human Mycotic Diseases. Springfield, Charles C. Thomas, 1975: 74-102.

246.   Top Cultures. Astaxanthin.
        http://www.phytochemicals.info/phytochemicals/astaxanthin.php
        Accessed 2007 Dec 29.

247.   Tripathy U, Yung GL, Kriett JM, Thistlethwaite PA, Kapelanski DP, Jamieson SW. Donor transfer of pulmonary coccidioidomycosis in lung transplantation. Ann Thorac Surg. 2002 Jan;73(1):306-8.

248.   Truett AA, Crum NF. Coccidioidomycosis of the prostate gland: two cases and a review of the literature. South Med J. 2004 Apr;97(4):419-22.

249.   University of Utah Department of Pathology. Pulmonary Pathology Case 7.
        http://www.path.utah.edu/casepath/PM%20Cases/PMCase7/ALL7.htm
        Accessed 2008 Feb 10.

250.   USDA. ARS Timeline.
        http://www.ars.usda.gov/is/timeline/1990chron.htm Accessed 2007 Jan 10.

251.   Usuki F, Yasutake A, Umehara F, Higuchi I. Beneficial effects of mild lifelong dietary restriction on skeletal muscle: prevention of age-related mitochondrial damage, morphological changes, and vulnerability to a chemical toxin. Acta Neuropathol (Berl). 2004 Jul;108(1):1-9. Epub 2004 Apr 17.

252.   Valdivia L, Nix D, Wright M, Lindberg E, Fagan T, Lieberman D, Stoffer T, Ampel NM, Galgiani JN. Coccidioidomycosis as a common cause of community-acquired pneumonia. Emerg Infect Dis. 2006 Jun;12(6):958-62.

253.   Valley Fever Center for Excellence. Frequently Asked Questions.
        http://www.vfce.arizona.edu/FAQ.htm Accessed 2008 Apr 15.

254.   Walsh TJ, Groll AH. Emerging fungal pathogens: evolving challenges to immunocompromised patients for the twenty-first century. Transpl Infect Dis. 1999 Dec;1(4):247-61.

255.   Washington State Department of Health. Fungus- and Tick-borne Diseases can be Severe. EpiTrends 2003 Jan;8(1):2.
        http://www.doh.wa.gov/Publicat/EpiTrends/03_EpiTrends/EpiTrendsJan03rev.pdf Accessed 2007 Nov 15.

256.   WebMD Drug Reference. www.webmd.com Accessed 2004 May 27.

257.   Werner SB, Vugia DJ, Duffey P, Williamson J, Bissell S, Jackson RJ, Rutherford GW. California Department of Health Services' Policy Statement on Coccidioidomycosis. In: Einstein HE, Catanzaro A, eds. Coccidioidomycosis. Proceedings of the 5th International Conference on Coccidioidomycosis. Stanford University, 24-27 August, 1994. Washington, DC. National Foundation for Infectious Diseases; 1996: 363-372.

258. Williams FM, Markides V, Edgeworth J, Williams AJ. Reactivation of coccidioidomycosis in a fit American visitor. Thorax. 1998 Sep;53(9):811-2.

259. Winn WA. The clinical development and management of coccidioidomycosis. In Ferguson MS, ed. Proceedings of Symposium on Coccidioidomycosis. Atlanta, Public Health Service Publication No. 575, 1957: 10-24.

260. Winter WG Jr, Larson RK, Honeggar MM, Jacobsen DT, Pappagianis D, Huntington RW Jr. Coccidioidal arthritis and its treatment. J Bone Joint Surg Am. 1975; 57:1152-1157. Cited in: Holley K, Muldoon M, Tasker S. Coccidioides immitis osteomyelitis: a case series review. Orthopedics 2002 Aug;25(8):827-31, 831-2.

261. Woods CW, McRill C, Plikaytis BD, Rosenstein NE, Mosley D, Boyd D, England B, Perkins BA, Ampel NM, Hajjeh RA. Coccidioidomycosis in human immunodeficiency virus-infected persons in Arizona, 1994-1997: incidence, risk factors, and prevention. J Infect Dis. 2000 Apr;181(4):1428-34.

262. Wright PW, Pappagianis D, Wilson M, Louro A, Moser SA, Komatsu K, Pappas PG. Donor-related coccidioidomycosis in organ transplant recipients. Clin Infect Dis. 2003 Nov 1;37(9):1265-9.

263. Wu J, Linscott AJ, Oberle A, Fowler M. Pathology case of the month. Occupational hazard? Coccidioidomycosis (Coccidioides immitis). J La State Med Soc. 2003 Jul-Aug;155(4):187-8.

264. Wu X, Gu L, Holden J, Haytowitz DB, Gebhardt SE, Beecher G, Prior RL. Development of a database for total antioxidant capacity in foods: a preliminary study. Papers from the Joint Meeting of the 5th International Food Data Conference and the 27th US National Nutrient Databank Conference. Vol 17, Issues 3-4, Jun-Aug 2004, 407-422, Accessed at http://www.nal.usda.gov/fnic/foodcomp/Data/Other/jfca17_407-422.pdf 2007 Jan 28.

265. Yin Y, Fu W, Fu M, He G, Traore L. The immune effects of edible fungus polysaccharides compounds in mice. Asia Pac J Clin Nutr. 2007;16 Suppl 1:258-60.

266. Yorgin PD, Rewari M, al-Uzri AY, Theodorou AA, Scott KM, Barton LL. Coccidioidomycosis in adolescents with lupus nephritis. Pediatr Nephrol. 2001 Jan;16(1):77-81.

267. Zheng R, Jie S, Hanchuan D, Moucheng W. Characterization and immunomodulating activities of polysaccharide from Lentinus edodes. Int Immunopharmacol. 2005 May;5(5):811-20. Epub 2004 Dec 2.

268. Zhou X, Lin J, Yin Y, Zhao J, Sun X, Tang K. Ganodermataceae: natural products and their related pharmacological functions. Am J Chin Med. 2007;35(4):559-74.

Index of Drugs and Tests

Amphotericin B, 103,104-7
  comparison with azole
    drugs, 110-1
  Fungizone formulation,
    106
  lipid formulations, 106
  user testimonials, 61, 143,
    151, 156, 162,163, 175
Biopsies, 96-7
  and lung cancer, 42, 98
  patient testimonials, 52,
    153, 159, 160, 166
Bronchoscopy 98
  patient testimonials 164,
    166
Cancidas. See *caspofungin*.
Caspofungin, 113
Complement fixation titer,
    89-90
  accuracy of, 49, 78, 79-80,
    88-9, 96
  interpreting test results,
    94, 95
Computed tomography. See
  CT scan.
CT scan, 99
  radiation dangers, 70-2
Cultures, 96-8
  picture of cultured
    spherules, 9
Diflucan. See *fluconazole*.
EIA Tests, 90, 92, 95, 96

ELISA Tests, 90-2, 95
Eosinophil count tests, 100
Erythrocyte sedimentation
  rate, 99-100
ESR. See *erythrocyte
  sedimentation rate*.
Fluconazole, 110-11
  user testimonials, 53, 58,
    60, 159, 161, 163, 164
  pet owners' experiences,
    138-9, 140, 141, 142, 144,
    145, 146-7
  comparison with
    amphotericin B, 111
  comparison with
    itraconazole, 109
  comparison with
    voriconazole, 112
False negative tests, 79-80,
  87-9
Fungizone, 106
  See also *amphotericin B*.
Immunodiffusion, 91-6
  qualitative
  immunodiffusion
    titer, 91.
Itraconazole, 109-10
  comparison with
    posaconazole, 111
  pet owners' experiences,
    138
  user testimonials 60, 153

Ketoconazole, 108-9
  comparisons with
    voriconazole and
    posaconazole, 113
  pet owners' experiences,
    138-140
Latex agglutination, 91, 93,
  94, 95
MRI, 99
  gadolinium based contrast
    agents, 72-74
Nikkomycin Z, 116, 179-80
Nizoral. See *ketoconazole*.
Noxafil. See *posaconazole*.
Posaconazole, 111-112
Qualitative immunodiffusion
  titer, 91.
Sed rate. See *erythrocyte
  sedimentation rate*.

Sporanox. See *itraconazole*.
Titer. See also *compliment
  fixation titer* and
  *immunodiffusion, qualitative
  immunodiffusion titer*.
Tube precipitin, 90, 93, 94,
  95
Voriconazole, 112-113
Vfend. See *voriconazole*.
Vaccines, 113-5.
  congressional support, 2
  UTSA vaccine, 115, 178
  support from Valley Fever
    Survivor, 178
  Valley Fever Vaccine
    Project, 114-5, 178
X-ray, 99
  reasons to keep copies, 76

About The Authors

Sharon Filip

As a Valley Fever Survivor, Sharon has dedicated her life to helping people that have contracted Valley Fever and warning those who have not. She and her son David created www.valleyfeversurvivor.com in 2002. It has become an advocacy organization to provide support for patients and to obtain funding for vaccine and cure projects.

Their web site has been visited by over 120 countries and territories around the world. Sharon receives e-mails from coast to coast and internationally from people and families affected by this disease. She has helped thousands of readers through e-mail and phone contact, and sometimes uses her years of experience as a professional hypnotherapist to help those who suffer from depression because of their Valley Fever. Sharon has been a motivational speaker, lecturer, and educator for decades and applies these skills in her fight against Valley Fever.

David Filip

After his mother's Valley Fever infection in 2001, David Filip dedicated his life to in-depth research of medical journals and every important conference on this subject. He has also been in telephone and e-mail contact with leading researchers and hundreds of Valley Fever Survivors.

David has a BA degree in communications from the University of Washington and is a member of the New York Academy of Sciences. His extensive research and natural writing ability enabled him to make www.valleyfeversurvivor.com the only comprehensive, up-to-date web site available on this disease. By bringing the medical, military, historical, and personal facets of Valley Fever together, David's knowledge and expertise "connects the dots" in ways that bring the complete scope of the Valley Fever epidemic to light.

David Filip is also a technical writer, a black belt in Arnis, and a musician with music and sound effects appearing in video games and multimedia displays.

<u>Notes</u>

CPSIA information can be obtained at www.ICGtesting.com
Printed in the USA
239271LV00004B/8/P